RECOVERY
FROM SEXUAL ADDICTION:
A MAN'S GUIDE

RECOVERY
FROM SEXUAL ADDICTION:
A MAN'S GUIDE

Paul Becker, LPC

authorHOUSE®

AuthorHouse™
1663 Liberty Drive
Bloomington, IN 47403
www.authorhouse.com
Phone: 1-800-839-8640

Published by AuthorHouse   05/03/2012

ISBN: 978-1-4685-7717-4 (sc)
ISBN: 978-1-4685-7716-7 (e)

Table of Contents

Acknowledgments

To those who shared their stories—and only you know who you are—you will be indispensable to those who will benefit from sharing your journey.

I would like to thank and acknowledge Sherry Hart, Patricia Doane, and Dr. Ann Johnson who read drafts and made valuable and appreciated contributions to this endeavor.

God bless you all.

Other books by Paul Becker, LPC

Letters from Paul

In Search of Recovery: A Christian Man's Guide

In Search of Recovery Workbook: A Christian Man's Guide

In Search of Recovery: Clinical Guide

Why Is My Partner Sexually Addicted? Insight women Need

Recovery From Sexual Addiction: A Man's Workbook

This book, *Recovery From Sexual Addiction: A Man's Guide*, is a revised edition and replaces, *In Search of Recovery: A Christian Man's Guide. Recovery From Sexual Addiction: A Man's Guide,* adds substantial new material.

The book, *Recovery From Sexual Addiction: A Man's Workbook*, is a revised edition and replaces, *In Search of Recovery Workbook: A Christian Man's Guide.*

Quotations or concepts from the book *Facing the Shadow: Starting Sexual and Relationship Recovery,* are used or reprinted with permission of Dr. Patrick Carnes and Gentle Path Press.

Quotations or concepts from the book, *Contrary to Love: Helping the Sexual Addict,* are used or reprinted with permission of Dr. Patrick Carnes and the Hazelden Foundation.

Quotations or concepts from the book, *Don't Call it Love: Recovery from Sexual Addiction,* and *Out of the Shadows: Understanding Sexual Addiction* are used or reprinted with permission of Dr. Patrick Carnes.

Preface

There was a time when I thought I was on my way to hell. I believed, of all of the people on earth who deserved God's love, I was not one of them. How could God love a man who turned His very special gift, human sexuality, into tragedy? Unwanted sexual behavior was a part of my life. I vowed to change my behavior but failed every promise. Hope eluded me.

In the early eighties my employer sent me to a prestigious university. While there, I scoured the many libraries connected with the university to find information and help on what was called sexual addiction. I found very little information outside of clinical case studies of aberrant sexual behavior. The information I found only darkened my cloud of shame.

While at school, I entered therapy with a noted psychologist. Unfortunately, he too knew little about sexual addiction. Although I did not realize it at the time, the Lord was at my side. He gave me an important insight that began my recovery journey. I realized that my first step was to gain control over my mind and to end sexual thinking and fantasy. This insight, and many more to follow, helped me turn addiction into recovery. Later, I was fortunate to find a therapist who helped me understand the origin of my sexual addiction and the adult choices I could now make.

Perhaps you too find yourself in a wasteland of hopelessness. Perhaps you wonder if you are worthy of God's love. Perhaps you don't know where to turn. Perhaps you have been led to this book. I felt called to write this book for you—so you too can change addiction into recovery.

The journey to sexual sobriety takes time. Expect it. I asked my therapist when sexual temptation will end. He smiled and said, "At the moment of death. However," he said, "you will note change. At a future Thanksgiving dinner you will reflect back and see that you have come a long way. You will realize that your investment in sobriety has loosened the bounds of addiction. You will realize, even though temptation has not ended, sexual addiction no longer holds you captive." Is it time to begin your journey?

The lies that sexually addicted men tell themselves are many. Some of my lies were, "Nobody will find out," and, "I am really not hurting anybody." Lies keep us from accepting the help we need. They are the excuses used to justify our need to continue sexually addictive behavior. What lies are you telling yourself to justify continuing your behavior? Do any of these lies seem familiar?

- My viewing pornography does not impact my marriage.

- All the men I know view pornography and it doesn't seem be a problem for them.

- Masturbation is healthy.

- I need my sexual fantasy to relieve my anxiety.

- My extramarital affair is my business and besides nobody will find out.

- So what if I mentally undress a woman. Who will know?

- I have a high libido and need more sex then I get in my marriage.

- The only way I relax is by viewing pornography.

- I can stop whenever I want to.

The lies sexually addicted men believe create a barrier to seeking help. Every rationalization that keeps a sexually addicted man from accepting help is a **bold face lie**. I know, I told many lies before I realized that my behavior had to change. Is it time for you to give up your lies and accept help?

It is hard for a sexually addicted man to visualize what life will be like further down the recovery road. I like to view the road as one with "potholes." Early on in the recovery journey the potholes are quite large and each time we fall into one of them we need the helping hand of a counselor or accountability partner to pull us back onto the road. As time goes by, climbing out of the pothole requires less help. Eventually, we see the potholes coming and are able to navigate around them or jump over them. While the potholes continue during our journey, the day comes when they are no longer big enough to cause us difficulty. Are you ready to begin the journey to sexual sobriety?

Introduction

Is this book for me? Why should I read this book?

- Have you tried to stop your unwanted sexual behavior and found your efforts have been unsuccessful?

- Is your sexual behavior followed by feelings of guilt and shame? Are you are tired of feeling guilty and ashamed?

- Have you wondered whether you need to do something about your sexual behavior? Do you need help to answer that question?

- Do you keep your sexual activity a secret from your spouse, children, and friends? Are you reluctant to ask for help? Do you feel embarrassed to talk about your unwanted sexual behavior?

- Do you think you are betraying your spouse, children, friends, and family by engaging in sexual behavior?

- Do you feel a distancing between God and yourself as a result of your sexual behavior?

- Do you allow sexual thinking and fantasy to occupy significant parts of your day?

- Have you wondered why sex has become a dominating factor in your life?

If so, this book is for you! It will begin your journey to a healthy sexual life.

How can this book help me?

You engage in unwanted sexual behavior, but do you know why? You will learn about the characteristics of sexual addiction. You will learn why you struggle with repetitive sexual behavior. You will obtain insights into other men's journeys—what has helped them to address their unwanted sexual behavior. You will learn there is hope as well as ways to change your behavior. You can restore your relationship with the Lord.

Paul Becker, LPC

What this book is not

Although this book is intended to give its readers insights into unwanted sexual behavior, it is not intended as a substitute for counseling, nor is it a substitute for a Twelve Step program. Freedom from unwanted sexual behavior often requires the aid of a counselor or therapist. A therapist can help you see beyond your blind spots and guide you on your recovery journey. Unaided efforts will likely fail and thus delay recovery.

What is recovery? Is it a cure?

The concept of "cure" connotes a full restoration to health. It may not be possible to eliminate all unwanted sexual urges. Although sexual thoughts and temptations may continue, it is very possible to reach a stage where you no longer act on them. If that is a cure, so be it. For most men the word recovery is a more apt descriptor. It conveys the sense of a journey—one that continues throughout life. In Twelve Step programs addicts are encouraged to take their recovery "one day at a time." Emphasis is on the present, not the future.

If I need counseling or therapy anyway, why read this book?

Recovery involves choices that are best made after gaining an understanding of the dynamics underlying each choice. Changing thinking patterns requires an understanding of the reasons why they ought to change. Recovery begins with enlightenment or gaining a greater awareness of one's self. Seek to know how and why unwanted sexual behavior became part of your life and why it continues despite your wanting to stop. This book will begin the process of enlightenment. It will raise your awareness so that, in time, your choices will become clearer and you will be empowered to exercise new choices that change the dance.

Is sexual addiction a disease?

The mental health profession's guide for diagnosing mental illness is the *Diagnostic Statistical Manual* (DSM IV). The DSM IV devotes a chapter to sexual and gender identity disorders. The closest the DSM IV comes to discussing sexual addiction is *Paraphilias*.

The Paraphilias are characterized by recurrent, intense sexual urges, fantasies, or behaviors that involve unusual objects, activities, or situations and cause clinically significant distress or impairment in social, occupational, or other important areas of functioning. The Paraphilias include Exhibitionism, Fetishism, Frotteurism, Pedophilia, Sexual Masochism, Sexual Sadism, Transvestic Fetishism, Voyeurism, and Paraphilia Not Otherwise Specified. (American Psychiatric Association, 2000)

Each of these above characteristics and types of behavior is presented in this book.

At this time the DSM IV does not address addiction to pornography, compulsive masturbation, sexual affairs, and compulsive use of massage parlors, prostitution, or online sex, etc., as mental health illnesses. Nevertheless, trouble with these issues brings the majority of men to seek help. Sexual behaviors in this sense, while not classified as a mental illness, cause the addicted man and his family much pain.

Sexual addiction has antisocial implications similar to excessive alcohol or drug use. Like alcohol or drug use, sexual addiction becomes the most important driving force in an addict's life. Use grows to the point of compulsive repetition and the addict is no longer able to change behavior except for short periods of time.

For compulsive masturbation, the most common unwanted sexual behavior, the attachment is more insidious than alcohol. For example, an alcoholic who needs a drink must make arrangements to procure alcohol and have it available. This requires some preplanning. The sexually addicted man carries his drink with him in his brain and genitals. His brain and genitals are always available. Desire and place are all that is needed. The memory is capable of storing volumes of sexually stimulating material, making each man a walking sexual brewery and bar.

While many forms of unwanted sexual behavior are sometimes classified as healthy by some, that same behavior causes many men significant distress. It causes them to experience less than full lives.

Note: This book and its predecessor have been a work in progress for several years and contains a synthesis of material from multiple sources that I have used in sexual addiction counseling. However, all names of men used in vignettes have been changed. This book, while primarily for men struggling with sex addiction, may also provide valuable insights to women about male sexual addiction. However, a better choice for women would be the book: *Why Is My Partner Sexually Addicted?* (Can be purchased on-line . . . just type the title into your browser.)

Real knowledge is to know the extent of one's ignorance.

Confucius

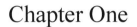

Chapter One

What is Sexual Addiction?

Ben's story

Ben talked about his sex life with his wife Betty. He believed he was entitled to sex at least four or five times a week. He was angry with Betty when she did not meet his needs. She told Ben there was more to sex than "slam bam, thank you Ma'am." To Ben it was simple. He was the head of the household, he worked very hard, he was entitled to sex when he wanted it, and it was Betty's job to be there for him. How could she not understand his needs?

Ben spent many hours a week, often daily, on the Internet searching for more and more stimulating pornography. When he got aroused, he thought that Betty was his outlet. If Betty declined to meet his needs, Ben masturbated. After masturbating, he felt shame and guilt, and those feelings made him angrier with Betty. They argued about sex daily.

Ben and Betty were living a crisis in their marriage and the crisis was not how frequently Ben wanted sex. The crisis was built on the many misconceptions of the true meaning of marital relations. It was over the role of sexual activity. It was over Ben's sexual addiction to pornography, and, yes, Betty was right, sex should be far more than "slam bam, thank you Ma'am."

In therapy, Ben began to peel the layers of his many misconceptions related to sexual behavior. He saw that he was preoccupied with sex—any way he could get it. He began to understand that sex had taken over his life. He estimated that he thought about sex somewhere between a third and half of the day, and he realized he was powerless over pornography—he needed his "fix" many times a week. Ben knew he was sexually addicted and his life had become miserable.

In today's world many men are sexually addicted. When lecturing to a male audience, a therapist often suggests that if they look to the man on their left and to the man on their right, there is a high likelihood that one of the two will deal with sexual addiction some time during his life. Are you a man who needs to deal with sexual addiction? Are you beginning to understand that sexual thinking and sexual activity are claiming too much of your life?

This book assumes you are engaging in unwanted sexual behavior. You may not have made the decision that your sexual behavior is unwanted. For many reasons, men often think they are justified in maintaining their sexual behavior or believe their behavior is normal, "all men do it." The first step is to make a decision: Is your sexual behavior wanted or unwanted? If your sexual behavior is wanted, is it getting you the life you really want?

Let's begin by learning the attributes of sexual addiction. Later we will name and define commonly accepted types of unwanted sexual behavior. We will also name the Devil and raise your awareness of the underlying factors that lead to sexual addiction.

What is Addiction?

> In his book, *Bradshaw on: The Family*, John Bradshaw (1988), defines addiction as "any pathological relationship with any mood-altering experience that has life-damaging consequences."

Further, he states:

> Pathological implies a delusional quality to the relationship. Delusion and denial are the essence of addictive compulsive behavior. In denial one denies what one is doing is really harmful, either to self or others. In delusion we believe that what is happening is not happening in spite of the facts.

Sexually addictive behavior or what this book calls acting out, alters mood. An orgasm is a very powerful mood-altering experience, which affects a physical as well as a mental change. Both changes are highly pleasurable. God made us to enjoy the climax of sexual stimulation. For the addict, the mood-altering experience is a form of self-medication employed in order to temporarily forget, cover up, hide, ignore, or otherwise not deal with underlying painful life conditions. However, for the addict, the underlying painful condition is not altered by orgasm; thus, he compulsively repeats the act to escape reality.

Addicts often delude themselves by focusing on frequency. Mark picked up women at bars. He confided, "I really have my addiction under control. I only slip every few months." Mark asserted that frequency was the defining point to addiction. Mark, in fact, was in denial and had a serious addiction—one that eventually cost him his job and marriage.

Aside from legal aspects, that which is life-damaging is unique to each person's internal code of values. Masturbation is a case in point. Many believe that masturbation is a healthy way of relieving sexual tension. For others it is a betrayal of self—a secret activity that leads to feelings of shame and guilt. Some married men believe sexually acting out alone is a betrayal of the marriage contract.

Life-damaging consequences are experienced when sexual addiction (that is, unwanted sexual activity, fantasy, or sexual thinking) begins to interfere with work, relationships, social activities, home life, and finances. Men often report that sexual thinking and masturbation occupy several hours of the day.

Although the focus here is on unwanted sexual behavior, most addicts have multiple addictions. Some are more harmful than others. For example, when a person is co-addicted to alcohol and unwanted sexual behavior, both addictions have life-damaging consequences. Both need to be addressed from the beginning. When a person is co-addicted to work (workaholic) and unwanted sexual behavior, the addiction to work usually does not have life-damaging consequences in the short run. The unwanted sexual behavior is the most damaging and needs to be addressed first. However, in therapy a connection between the two addictions may be found.

In *Treating Sexual Shame: A New Map for Overcoming Dysfunction, Abuse, and Addiction*, Anne Stirling Hastings (1998) says, "Fear of intimacy, sexual and otherwise, is a major cause of sexual addiction." Sexually addicted men are isolated; non-sexual intimacy is for most a mystery. For the addict, intimacy equals sex. Sex is the addict's primary need.

What Are the Common Characteristics of Unwanted Sexual Behavior?

Multiple practices

Unwanted sexual behavior includes a large number of sexual practices. Later in this chapter we will list and define many of these practices. It is common to find men who engage in more than one practice. It is also common for a man to begin with one type of unwanted sexual behavior and progress into others over time. For example, young people often find masturbation attractive as they discover the nature of their sexuality. At some point a youth may discover pornography and begin to use it as a stimulant. Later in life, paper pornography may lead to Internet pornography and eventually paying for online sex.

Obsession

The greatest need of a sexually addicted man is to experience his form of acting out, whether it is pornography and masturbation, multiple affairs, or any other acting-out behavior. Left unchecked the addict dedicates much of his day to repeating the behaviors that give him significant pleasure or shields him from experiencing depressed mood, anxiety, and other social or mental health problems.

The addict is obsessed with the filling his needs. For example, an addict, after his spouse has retired for the night, may spend many hours in search of explicit and tantalizing images or videos on the Internet. His obsession is to find the perfect image or video that matches his unique mental concept of sexual perfection. However, he continually searches for his version of the Holy Grail without success. Each successive image, while stimulating, is never the end of the search. When his search leads to arousal so that orgasm follows, he has completed most of one sex addiction cycle. The cycle continues following orgasm during which he feels guilt and shame. During this phase of the cycle the addict tells himself he does not plan to repeat this behavior, but his obsession leads him to repeat it time and again.

Compulsive-powerlessness

Ultimately the sexually addicted man forfeits his God given gift of free will. His addiction forms such a choke hold that he no longer has the ability to choose to refrain from his sexual behavior. Overtime, his acting out becomes a habitual repetition of behaviors that lead to orgasm. His normal control mechanisms become impaired or disabled. He develops a psychological dependence based on the flow of brain chemicals, endorphin and adrenaline. The hyper flow of these chemicals creates neuron pathways which take prominence in determining his behavior. In other words, his brain forms roadways to facilitate the onset of feelings, thinking, and activities which lead to the psychological and physical high associated with orgasm

Ted's story

Ted came to counseling after having visited a house of ill repute in a local city. While he expressed considerable remorse for having fallen, he was particularly concerned that he might have been exposed to a venereal disease. He spent most of the session talking about how sorry he was that he had befallen God's trust. Because of finances, Ted scheduled his next counseling appointment for a month later. Ted did not return for his second session. In a follow-up telephone conversation, Ted declared that he was not a sexually addicted man. He said he had his behavior under control and that he would not fall again. About six months later Ted revisited the same house of ill repute. Ted's acting-out cycle was a lengthy one and he fell to a common misunderstanding that sexually addicted men repeat their behaviors daily or at least weekly. Some addicts, in fact, are not daily users of sexual stimulation, but engage in sporadic binges. Ted compulsively repeated his behavior just as a man who repeats his behavior frequently. Sex addicted men invariably feel compelled to repeat their behavior. They are powerless to "take or leave" their sexual behaviors.

Some in the mental health field feel that there is no such disorder as sexual addiction. They hold that a selective part of the male population is born with hyper sexuality. The reality is that a sexually addicted man does not enjoy sex any more or less than the average male. Healthy sexual relations are the mutual expression of love that ultimately results in intercourse. Sexual addictive behavior is not about love. It is about achieving orgasm. Sexual addicts are compelled to act out sexually notwithstanding their greater or lesser biological hyper sexuality.

Practices become unmanageable

What began as an occasional practice may increase to the point where one becomes powerless to stop. All the best intentions or pledges to stop become a long series of failed intentions. The unwanted sexual practice becomes part of a man's life. He is able to give up the practices only for short intervals. Eventually the practices become unmanageable and life-damaging consequences follow.

Carnes (1994) says it this way:

> Perhaps the best test of the presence of an addiction is its unmanageability. The therapist makes a thorough effort to *search for "out of control" behavior*. Chaos, which results from the addict's pursuit of the addiction scenario, provides many clues to the internal conflict that the addict experiences due to distorted priorities. Perhaps the surest sign is the addict repeatedly makes efforts to stop and fails, despite the obvious consequences of the behavior. Sometimes these efforts to control takes the form of dramatic changes—changing jobs, location, and even spouses—but to no avail. Tapping into the desire to quit is key to the assessment and also recovery. If it is an addiction, this desire is likely buried under layers of shame and impaired thinking.

For some men, the build up and subsequent orgasm is not designed to reap sexual pleasure but to ward off negative feelings. A successful businessman had difficulty coping with stress. Doubt that his business decisions were correct or would make him money caused him high levels of distress. He developed daily anxiety that was very painful to him. He learned at some point that if he masturbated, the anxiety level drops for a period of time. Following masturbation the reduced level of anxiety lasted but a few hours and he then needed to repeat his masturbation. He found himself masturbating four and five times a day, not for pleasure, but simply to reduce anxiety. His life became unmanageable because he felt that masturbation was the only way for him to relieve his anxiety. Despite advice to the contrary, he felt only weak men took anti-anxiety medication. This man came to counseling not to deal with his anxiety but because he could no longer perform in the marital bed. His wife told him to seek help or his alimony payments would be extraordinary. In counseling he and his counselor dealt with his underlying anxiety disorder and his sexual addiction behavior ended. His life became manageable once again.

A characteristic of unmanageability is the risk that sexually addicted men take. Joe was an assistant pastor at a local church. One day his church-issued laptop froze. He turned the laptop over to their IT contractor. The IT contractor discovered that the hard disk was full of pornography and there was no storage memory left. The IT contractor disclosed his discovery to the pastor. Joe and his pastor had a long discussion about Joe finding employment elsewhere. Joe risked his employment, his marriage, and his relationship with the Lord to satisfy his sexual needs. The good news is that Joe and his pastor agreed Joe would enter counseling. A long-term benefit was that Joe could share knowledge of his sexual addiction with his youth and his young men's groups. His words relayed authenticity to the young men in his church because he dealt with sexual temptation as they did. He was able to bond with men who needed to know that clergy are real people and have the same failings.

Another characteristic of unmanageability is the tendency of sexually addicted men to procrastinate. Almost by definition sexually addicted men have low self-esteem and negative feelings about their ability to produce a successful product. Because they fear failure, which would confirm their feelings of worthlessness, sexually addicted men have a propensity to delay work assignments until they have no other choice. Most sexually addicted men are bright and their failure to produce is not due to a lack of intelligence or skill. Nevertheless, procrastination is a manifestation of an unmanageable life.

Another example of an unmanageable life is the ability for the sexually addicted man to tell himself lies and actually believe his lies. While this subject will be explored later in the book, a short example is given here to illustrate. Seth knew full well that going on his computer late at night was the first step toward acting out. In a group program, he shared that he planned to change his approach to the use of his computer. Seth said he would no longer use his computer after his wife went on to bed. At the next session he told the group what happened. He said he had no intention of going to any pornographic web sites when he turned on the computer to check his e-mail. However, he said once he turned on his computer it was like going down a slippery slope. He checked e-mail, went to a sports page, saw an attractive image of a singer, checked-out the singer's web page, and went on to view pornography. He believed the lie that late at night he could turn on his computer and not end up in pornography.

The behavior is unmanageable when it becomes a conditioned response. Pavlov conditioned a dog to respond to a trigger in the form of a bell. For example, when conditioned, the addict will respond to turning on his computer as a trigger that leads to acting out.

Tolerance

Each time a man replays a sexual fantasy in his brain, he strengthens the image in his sexual mental file cabinet. He becomes more bonded to the draw of the image. Sexually addicted men engage in escalating patterns of sexual behavior despite increasingly negative consequences.

Classic tolerance for the sexually addicted man is the need to experience ever increasing higher levels of stimulation. Some men can no longer get aroused by their earlier sexual practices. Jeff visited massage parlors. He continually sought out new establishments in hopes that he would find a masseuse with a new way of stimulating his arousal. After having tried every massage parlor in his city he decided that he would see if a prostitute could improve upon his experiences with masseuses. He continued to look for more and better sexual encounters even trying sexual sadism. Massage parlors or prostitutes no longer did it for him.

Progression

Progression, like tolerance, leads men to seek more stimulating images or experiences.

Ewald (2003) says:

> Sexual addiction is progressive and it rarely gets better. Over time it gets more frequent and more extreme. At other times when it seems under control, the addict is merely engaging in one of the common traits of the disease process in which he switches from sexual release to the control of it. The control phase inevitably breaks down over time and the addict is back in the behavior again, despite his promise to himself or others never to do it again. When the ecstasy of the release is spent, the addict will feel remorse at his failure and will switch back to another "white knuckle" period of abstaining from the behavior until his resolve weakens again.

Almost universally men in recovery groups talk about how their search for more stimulating pornographic images has taken them to places that they never expected they would go. While they started with viewing women in conventional sex, they often progressed to more bizarre images and videos. Only rarely does a man who initially enjoys adult sexual images, progresses to view child pornography.

Withdrawal

Psychological withdrawal symptoms accompany efforts to stop or cut back on one's behavior. Such symptoms include discomfort, irritability or restlessness.

The most important withdrawal symptom is the fear of losing one's most cherished friend. Since, for most men, sexual addiction began in childhood, the number of years they have been in relationship with their addiction usually spans decades. The pleasurable experience from orgasm has been fully encoded in their brains over the years. The brain has continued to demand that the addict provide it with its run of adrenalin and endorphins. Giving up his cherished behaviors is like experiencing cold terror in the night. Men in therapy talk about this loss. It is not an easy challenge. At the beginning of the commitment to change one's behavior, the victories may be counted in minutes or hours and perhaps a week. Each victory becomes a milestone. Each milestone becomes an investment in sobriety.

Life-damaging consequences

Isolation is a primary life-changing consequence. Rarely is a man proud of his unwanted sexual behavior. Thus, he finds he cannot talk about it within his normal support system (his wife, friends, or relatives). He withdraws in fear that he will be judged as a bad person—someone with a problem he no longer can control. Other consequences may include self-loathing, depression, anxiety, and anger. He may find that his relationships are damaged, particularly those with his family and his God. Shame and guilt become constant companions. Feelings of loss of control are painful and may yield to despair and a pervasive feeling of hopelessness.

Change in a life focus

Sexual behavior becomes a primary motivator, a primal need. Wanted or unwanted sexual behavior becomes so time consuming that it takes precedence over sleep, work, and healthy recreational activities. Paying for the cost of sex may take precedence over other family living expenses. Obtaining sexual gratification becomes so energy consuming that it displaces day-to-day functions and pleasures. For example, a man named Henry quipped, "I love to hear a woman talk dirty. I have a list of numbers that I call." Henry came to counseling when his credit card debt exceeded $20,000 due to phone sex. For Henry, life was defined by looking forward each day to engaging in phone sex.

Sex addiction cycle and rituals

A man caught up in unwanted sexual behavior will repeat one or more patterns of acting out. A man addicted to prostitution will cruise the streets even though he tells himself that he is just going to the store. He engages in a repetitive ritual that always gets him to the same place—acting out. In Chapter 3, the sex addiction cycle and acting out rituals will be fully explored.

Denial

Invariably the man caught in a pattern of repetitive unwanted sex will develop illogical thinking to justify his behavior. Frequently heard excuses include:

- I am not hurting anybody.

- I deserve a little happiness in my life.

- I plan to quit, but I am under stress now.

- I have a much higher libido than others I know and I need this outlet.

- I can control this when I want to. I don't need help.

- It only happens every once in awhile.

- How else am I going to relieve my tremendous sexual tension?

Addicted men actually believe their lies and often avoid getting the help they need. It is rare for anyone working on his or her own to overcome addiction.

Unwanted Sexual Behaviors Found in the DSM IV

The authority on definitions for counselors and therapists is the *Diagnostic and Statistical Manual of Mental Disorders* (DSM IV). This guidebook classifies mental disorders and establishes common definitions and diagnostic standards for mental health specialists, insurance processing, and statistical analysis. It is the product of much research and study and represents the American Psychiatric Association's guidance to the mental health community at large.

The DSM IV classifies only a small proportion of what are considered unwanted sexual behaviors. But it is a good place to start. It defines unwanted sexual behaviors as paraphilias (American Psychiatric Association, 2000).

All paraphilias, according to the DSM IV, are characterized by reoccurring, intense sexual urges, sexual fantasies, or behaviors. Such fantasies, sexual urges, or behaviors must occur over at least a six-month period of time. They must also cause significant stress or impair one's social, occupational, or everyday functioning for a diagnosis to be made. There is also a sense of distress within these individuals. Typically, they recognize the symptoms as negatively impacting their lives but believe they are unable to control them.

Paraphilias included in the DSM IV include the following points.

Exhibitionism involves the surprise exposure of one's genitals to a stranger. Exposure may coincide with masturbation and a fantasy expectation that the stranger will become sexually aroused.

Fetishism involves the use of nonliving objects; for example, a woman's underpants, bras, or other worn apparel to achieve a state of arousal. The man frequently masturbates while holding, rubbing, or smelling the apparel. He may ask his sexual partner to wear the apparel during sexual encounters. The fetish is either preferred or required for sexual excitement.

Frotteurism involves touching and rubbing one's genitals against a non consenting person. The behavior generally occurs in crowded places to avoid arrest. The behavior may also involve fondling. During the act, the person usually fantasizes an exclusive, caring relationship with the victim.

Pedophilia is characterized by sexual activity with a child, usually ages 13 or younger, or in the case of an adolescent, a child five years younger than the pedophile.

Masochism involves the act of being humiliated, beaten, bound, or otherwise made to suffer to enhance or achieve sexual excitement. In some cases the act is limited to a fantasy of being raped while being held or bound by others so that there is no possibility of escape. Sexual masochism may involve a wide range of devices to achieve the desired effect, including some that may cause death.

Sadism involves an act in which the individual derives sexual excitement from the psychological or physical suffering, including humiliation, of the victim. The partner may or may not be consenting. Sadism may involve a wide range of behaviors and devices to achieve the desired effect.

Transvestic fetishism involves heterosexual males dressing in female clothes (cross-dressing) to produce or enhance sexual arousal, usually without a real partner, but with the fantasy that they are the female partner. Women's garments are arousing primarily as symbols of the individual's femininity.

Voyeurism involves observing an unknowing and non consenting person, usually a stranger, who is naked or in the process of becoming unclothed and/ or engaging in sexual activity. The act of looking (peeping) is intended to produce sexual excitement and is usually accompanied by self-masturbation. Fantasies from such acts are used to fuel future masturbation.

Unwanted Sexual Behaviors Not Found in DSM IV

The following unwanted sexual behaviors are not included in the DSM IV but may likewise result in significant stress or impair one's social, occupational or everyday functioning.

Extramarital affairs involve single or multiple sexual relationships with partners outside the marriage that cause significant stress to the marriage relationship. Men often justify an affair because of a perception of unfulfilled expectations within the marriage. Swinging and wife swapping are aberrant forms of extramarital affairs that include the participation of both marriage partners.

Multiple or anonymous partners often involve homosexual relationships—frequently anonymous, situational, and intended to provide sexual experience. Homosexual encounters also may be habitual since they are repeated time and again with new partners. They are particularly dangerous to the parties if practiced without the protection of a condom because participants are exposed to sexually transmitted diseases and HIV.

Prostitution involves the solicitation and procurement of various types of sexual behavior from male or female escorts or prostitutes. Sexual massage involves the solicitation and procurement of sex, most often oral sex or masturbation, from a male or female who provides massages. In most cases those who seek such services have a problem with other sexual behaviors.

Sexual anorexia involves an obsessive state in which the physical, mental, and emotional tasks of avoiding sex dominate one's life. Preoccupation with the avoidance of sex may be used to mask or avoid one's life problems. The obsession can then become a way to cope with all stress and all life difficulties.

Compulsive sexual behaviors

Our society judges some sexual behaviors as reasonably normal. Among men, little stigma is attached to them. The concepts, "every male does it," or "it doesn't hurt anyone," or similar thinking is used to justify the behavior. What changes a behavior from acceptable to unacceptable is compulsivity. That is, the sexual activity is excessive and time consuming; interferes with a person's daily routine, work, or social functioning; continues despite diminished pleasure or gratification; places the individual at risk of physical harm; or have legal or personal consequences and leads to financial debt. Examples include:

Masturbation involves sexual self-stimulation, most commonly by touching, stroking, or massaging the penis, clitoris, or vagina until orgasm is achieved. Masturbation is the most common form of sexual addiction.

Pornography is any material that depicts or describes sexual function for the purpose of stimulating sexual arousal upon the part of the consumer.

Cybersex has as its common elements: use of a computer, Internet access, expected anonymity, and sexually provocative material to generate arousal followed most often by masturbation. Multiple venues exist such as visual images of real or graphically generated persons, interactive sex through a web cam, chat rooms, and e-mail. Cybersex is increasing at a high rate.

Phone sex has as its common element the use of a phone to talk or listen to a provocative repertoire to generate arousal followed, most often, by masturbation.

Underlying Factors of Sexual Addiction

Thinking is often analogous to an onion. Thinking is layered—each layer is nearer to the core of truth. Let's peel another layer of the onion to learn more about the underlying factors that play a significant role in the practice of unwanted sexual behavior or sexual addiction. There are many layers to the onion so please be patient as we peel one at a time.

The following material has its origin in *Contrary to Love: Healing the Sexual Addict,* by Patrick Carnes (1994). Carnes is a leading contemporary theorist on sexual addiction. He has worked with hospitals, treatment programs, private therapists, and community groups to develop a sexual addiction screening test. We will adapt his test to provide a forum for a discussion of underlying factors leading to the practice of unwanted sexual behaviors. If you answer yes to several of the following questions, you may have begun to peel that layer of the onion to understanding your behavior.

Were you sexually abused as a child or adolescent?

Carnes (1992) found that 81 percent of addicts he surveyed remember being abused sexually in some way as a child. The abuse may have been blatant or subtle. If you were exposed to age-inappropriate sexual activity or sexually explicit material, it may have created a lasting memory and desire to repeat the same behavior or a derivative of that behavior in adult life. The very fact that you are able to recall such age-inappropriate sexual activity or sexually explicit material affirms that it did affect you.

It is not uncommon for a child to react to sexual abuse by experiencing Post-Traumatic Stress Disorder (PTSD). When the abuse is extreme and child is sensitive the shock to the child's psyche can be devastating. Symptoms of PTSD can begin congruent with the abuse or show up later in life. Stress in adulthood can trigger PTSD symptoms related to childhood abuse.

Not all sexually abused children become addicts, but a large percentage of sex addicts were abused as children.

In Chapter 2 we will explore, in greater depth, the link between an early childhood sexual stimulation and sexually acting out as an adult.

Do you regularly purchase sexually explicit magazines?

Exposure to age-inappropriate sexually explicit material is a form of sexual abuse. A child instinctively knows that sexually explicit material is not passed around the dinner table. A child easily picks up on the experience of titillating feelings while viewing or reading sexually explicit pictures or stories. The material causes arousal in the child. The feeling of arousal is a new and a pleasurable experience—so much so that, as the child grows, he knows that a source of pleasure can be renewed by using pornography. A child exposed to pornography will often continue to seek out such material as a teenager and as an adult. For many, it becomes habitual.

Do you regularly pursue online pornography?

Although the Internet is a blessing from many points of view, men addicted to online pornography find the Internet a curse. The amount of pornography available online probably exceeds that which the Library of Congress could house. An addicted man will spend many hours trying to find satisfaction only to need to search for more stimulating images. Pornography can become a never-ending pursuit of new material. Visual stimulation from online pornography usually leads to masturbation.

Men tell themselves that what they are doing on their own computer is private and they will not be discovered. Nothing could be further from the truth. For several technical reasons, private computers record and store downloaded images. The computer also records Web sites visited. If the user is in an office environment that uses a centralized server, all online transactions will be recorded and stored. Internet service providers record sites visited and such information may be requested for law enforcement purposes. Being discovered in that online fish bowl often leads men to seek help. Family members frequently and inadvertently discover downloaded pornography that may lead back to a husband or child.

The possibility of getting caught is just one undesirable consequence. Men often find they waste many hours during the day, week, and month seeking online stimulation. The need to check out an old or new web site becomes compulsive and repetitive. Men instinctively know online sex is a poor substitute for marital relations. Feelings of guilt and shame frequently follow online and masturbation sessions. (Chapter 4 is devoted to a full exploration of the consequences of pornography)

Are you often preoccupied with sexual thoughts?

According to A.S. Hastings (1998), "Sexual fantasy is addictive when it is used to create a pleasant hum to make otherwise boring or distressing activities seem more appealing"

Preoccupation with sexual thoughts often begins in childhood with exposure to age-inappropriate sexual activity or sexually explicit material. The child learns that sexually explicit material leads to sexual fantasy and to pleasurable feelings—an escape from the daily stresses of life. Thus, preoccupation with sexual thoughts frequently begins at a young age and continues into adulthood.

In adulthood, men engage in various forms of sexual thinking. They frequently will have a favorite fantasy and return to it in the same way a child looks for a cookie to eat. Whenever feelings of distress or anxiety become unbearable, sexual thinking is the solution. When a man is sexually hungry, a sexual fantasy is the first cookie to soothe that hunger.

Sexually addicted men will see a person or image and store the visualization away for future processing. Such men, over time, reserve a part of their memory for sexually stimulating images. The memory is like an on-call secret sexual filing cabinet. When in need, they pull out a "sexual file" and review and examine the contents. The contents are often mentally embellished and, once enjoyed, stored for future use. Memories of past sexual encounters are often stored for future stimulation.

What is the problem? Don't all of us have sexual memories?

Yes, all humans who have engaged in sexual activities have memories of what happened—some good and some they wish they could forget. It is a matter of degree. It would be abnormal for a married man not to have sexual thoughts about his wife. The married addict processes fantasies well beyond any healthy fantasies related to his wife. The addict devotes many hours a day to sexual fantasy and does not stop with the processing of a sexual fantasy. A sexual fantasy or recalled memory is frequently the first step toward other unwanted sexual activity. Masturbation or other unwanted sexual behavior is often preceded by sexual fantasy.

Does your spouse/significant other ever worry or complain about your sexual behavior?

Although your judgment of acceptable sexual behavior may be cross wired, those around you may have a clearer view. If others express concern, consider that they love you enough to speak up. Perhaps it is time to ask a counselor to help you sort out the truth.

Can you stop your sexual behavior when you know it's inappropriate?

Sexual addiction behavior is obsessive or compulsive.

According to Hastings (1998):

> While (unwanted sexual) behaviors distract from healthy sexuality, they are only addictive if they are also obsessive or compulsive; in other words, if the person has difficulty interrupting thoughts about sex, searching for sex, or acting sexually. While sexual addiction recovery tends to focus on behaviors, the trance state can begin many hours or days before the sexual activity. This is the obsessive part of the addiction. The sexual act can be brief, and is often unsatisfying. Or it can go on for hours, to the point of damaging tissues of the penis or vagina. This is the compulsion.

Sexual thinking and sexual activities become requirements. They are no longer optional. A sexual addict needs his fix much the same way a drug addict does.

A fundamental tenet of any addiction is the difficulty of stopping. Those who have smoked can relate to pledges to stop only to have the pledge go up in smoke with the next cigarette. Have you ever heard a smoker answer the question, "Have you ever successfully quit smoking?"—"Yes, many times!" Sexual addiction is no different. In Chapter 2 we explore the reasons why.

Do you ever feel bad about your sexual behavior?

When a child is exposed to age-inappropriate sexual activity or sexually explicit material, the mind and body respond. First is curiosity and arousal (arousal in a child may be limited to a faster pulse rate, heart beat, and a mental rush). After the event is over most children recognize that the event was not normal. If secrecy surrounds the event, the child may feel a desire to keep the event secret. The abnormality of the event, as compared with normal play, often leads the child to feel shame and guilt. Children often think (incorrectly) they are responsible for the occurrence of an event. If a pattern of unwanted sexual behavior started in childhood and was accompanied by feelings of shame and guilt, guilt and shame will also accompany the repetition of unwanted sexual behavior in adulthood. In Chapter 2 we will explore how shame and guilt are factors in the addict's addiction cycle and the acting-out ritual.

Has sexual behavior ever created problems for you or your family?

Perhaps the number one reason men seek counseling for their unwanted sexual behavior is because their spouse discovered their behavior. You may be angry or very remorseful that you have been found out, but perhaps discovery is the only way you will take first recovery steps. Although you and your family may be in great pain, understand that pain is a significant motivator.

Do you worry about people finding out about this behavior?

Think back to the first time in childhood when you were exposed to age-inappropriate sexual activity or sexually explicit material. Did you run to your parents to report this new and exciting news? Chances are that your parents were the last people on earth you wanted to find out. You may have thought they would punish you or not believe you if they were told. In adulthood, it is also likely you are not proud of your behavior. You fear you will be chastised if you are found out. You may even fear you will have to give up your behavior if discovered. You may fear social, employment, marriage, or legal consequences. Are your fears legitimate? Perhaps, but it is also likely your family and friends will be more forgiving of you than you are of yourself.

Do you lead a double life?

Living a double life leads to feelings of loneliness and isolation. On the one hand, you want your family and friends to view you as an upstanding citizen, a person who is successfully tackling the challenges of life. On the other hand, you feel a sense of shame that you need to continually return to sexual stimulation, whether it is daily or every few weeks or months. This secret life is a constant reminder that you live a lie—a lie you fear will eventually be discovered.

Do you keep secrets about your sexual or romantic activities from those important to you?

Often, an early step in healing is disclosure. Disclosure to a clergy member or therapist is a beginning step. If you have not disclosed your behavior to family and friends, you may be wise first to consult a counselor. Your life will begin to change upon disclosure. In Chapter 9, the conditions of disclosure are presented.

Has your behavior ever emotionally hurt someone?

If you have been found out by a spouse or family member, it is likely that they have been hurt emotionally. Your spouse and family may feel betrayed, fear the loss of the family structure, or fear social and economic consequences. Their feelings may be very raw and it may take much time for them to heal. Requesting forgiveness and receiving forgiveness does not make emotional pain vanish. Trust is broken and it takes action and effort on your part to change offending behavior and a period of freedom from acting out to rebuild trust. It takes time and prayer to renew a trust. Forgiving yourself is also a necessary step, but unless you change your life you cannot expect to be forgiven by others.

In addition, when you were found out, it is likely only partial disclosure occurred. It is likely that you have more to disclose. Disclosure is best done with the help of a counselor. Full disclosure may be therapeutic for you, but it may cause emotional havoc to your loved ones. They will need the help of a therapist to understand the behavior you disclose, the underlying causes of the behavior, and possible recovery steps.

You are also hurt emotionally. Perhaps your behavior is rooted in abuse you experienced in childhood. You will require help to heal your emotional wounds as well.

Are any of your sexual activities against the law? (For example, sex with minors, exposure of genitals in public)

If your behavior is considered illegal, you will need to consult with an attorney and a counselor. If you have abused a child or aged person, the counselor will report your behavior to the authorities. They are required to do so by professional ethics and by law. Consider the damage done to your victim and take the steps necessary to end the abuse.

Have you ever felt degraded by your sexual activity?

For some, there is a psychological need to be humiliated or pained to achieve sexual stimulation. If you think your behaviors fall into the definition of sexual sadism or masochism, and you want to change your thinking and behavior, seek the help of a professional counselor who is trained to help men with these behaviors.

Do you feel depressed after having sex?

If you practice unwanted sexual behavior, think that the behavior is inappropriate, are concerned that you will be found out, and/or feel guilty or shamed for your behavior, it is a natural consequence to feel depressed after your engagement. In addition, sexually addicted men are often isolated from their families and have few friends. They often live in a state of low-grade depression. In Chapter 6 you will explore the three coordinates of sexual addiction—acting out, anger/anxiety, and depression.

Do you fear sexual intimacy? Do you avoid sex at all costs?

Extremes often cause problems. If you obsessively avoid sex to cope with stress, it is likely that stress is adversely affecting many aspects of your life. As with most forms of unwanted sexual behavior, counseling may help you to establish perspective as to the effectiveness of your behavior for getting what you need from life.

Do you frequently feel remorse, shame, or guilt after a sexual encounter?

When sexual behavior causes negative feelings, it is a sure sign that something is amiss. Sex is a precious gift from God. It is not intended to be the source of remorse, shame, or guilt. One's conscience is also a precious gift from God, and when it tells you that one gift is at odds with another, it is time to seek help.

Carnes (1992) describes the link between shame and sexually acting out:

> *Addictive sex* feels shameful. Often it is illicit, stolen, or exploitive. It compromises values and draws on fear to generate excitement. Addictive sex often reenacts childhood abuses, disconnecting one from self. A world of unreality is created, allowing self-destructive and dangerous behaviors. Based on conquest or power, it is seductive and dishonest. Serving to medicate and

kill pain, addictive sex becomes routine, grim, and joyless. A tough taskmaster, the addiction requires a double life and demands perfection.

Have you ever tried to limit or stop masturbating?

Is masturbation normal and a healthy thing to do? It is not hard to find literature and health practitioners who say, "Go for it." When masturbation becomes compulsive to the tune of multiple times a day or week, when you spend waking hours thinking about the next time, when you devote large amounts of time to the repetition of the event, when you develop masturbation rituals to enhance the effect, when you begin to wonder if this is the way you want to live your life, it is time to seek help. Masturbation is not healthy for everyone.

Masturbation in conjunction with Internet pornography is one of the leading reasons why men seek help. Internet pornography helps men to foster unwanted sexual behavior faster than any other form of media. In Chapter 4 both pornography and masturbation are addressed fully.

Do you lose your sense of identity or meaning in life without sex or a love relationship?

Carnes (2001) tells us that sex becomes the addict's greatest need. If sex defines you and life is not satisfying without it, you may have crossed the line into compulsion. You may also have other mental health issues that keep you focused on sex as your solution to the pain of ordinary life. In any case, if sex is your main goal in life, it is time to find out why.

Does your pursuit of sex or romantic relationships interfere with your spiritual development?

We humans have a conscience—an internal thermometer. At an elevated reading, our gut tells us that we are out of bounds. Conscience is a gift from the Creator. It helps us to experience guilt. Appropriate guilt can lead us to change behavior and, in the case of addiction, to find help. Just as a child knows that exposure to age-inappropriate sexual activity or sexually explicit material is not right, adults know when the practice of certain sexual behavior is not right and their adult conscience bothers them. Feeling bad about behavior and ourselves often affects our relationship with God. A right conscience is a blessing. On the other hand, when we despair over our weaknesses, the powers of evil have us where they want us. If you are not proud of your sexual behavior, it is the right time to seek guidance?

Insights into Sexual Addiction

Dan Morris (2012) has posted his sexual addiction insights on the Kavod web site.

His insights are reproduced here because they provide a good summary of the world of sexual addiction.

1. Sex addiction resembles other addictions.

2. Sex addicts use sex to self-medicate, to numb distressful emotions.

3. Repeated numbing of distressful emotions can result in depression.

4. Sex addicts, therefore, use sex as an antidepressant.

5. Sex addicts, because they use sex to avoid feeling distressful emotions, also avoid emotional intimacies in relationships.

6. Sex addicts can feel very lonely and isolated.

7. Sexual addiction can be fueled by sexual fantasies that are a replacement for real-life interaction.

8. Sex addicts spend an unfortunate amount of time in their heads, avoiding life.

9. Sex addicts are often not in the moment, not in the here and now.

10. Sexual addiction can be progressive in nature.

11. Sometimes the sex addict wants more and more sexual involvement.

12. Sometimes the sex addict becomes involved in sexual activity that is more and more depraved (ritualistic, rigid, without caring, hurtful).

13. Because of their shame and fear about being found out, the sex addict might keep his behaviors secret.

14. This kind of secret keeping creates shame and depression.

15. Recovery requires that an individual have a thought-out plan of action.

16. Recovery is about breaking the secrecy and isolation.

17. Recovery means recovering the ability to feel.

18. There are many paths to recovery.

19. Recovery means reconnecting to a power within and outside of oneself.

20. The addiction is not the same entity as the human being that is afflicted by it.

21. The addiction is like a parasite or virus that invades the host, living off of it. The addiction is mindless.

22. The human is mindful.

23. Recovery is the process of recovering intelligence.

24. The addiction's first task is to cause the human host to forget.

25. Forgetting healthy directions leaves the human vulnerable.

26. A plan to abstain is a comprehensive plan that maps one's directions throughout the day and night.

27. We use other humans to keep us accountable to ourselves and others.

28. Recovery is developing caring, supportive relationships.

29. In these relationships there is safety to speak the truth.

**Our pain is the breaking of the shell that
encloses your understanding.**

Kahlil Gibran

Chapter Two

Why Me?

Did you wake up one day and decide that you wanted to be a sex addict? Did you think through the alternatives and say to yourself, "I would enjoy life more if sex was my primary need in life?"

You probably replied, "Of course not!" You are right; chances are you never consciously chose to become sexually addicted.

How did it happen? For nine out of ten men who become sexually addicted, the addiction had its beginnings in childhood.

Model One—Sexual Addiction Has its Origin in Late Teen Years or Early Twenties

For one in ten men who become sexually addicted, the addiction had its origin in late teen years or early twenties. These men grew up in a sexually sterile environment. Nothing sexual was ever mentioned or discussed in his home. His parents and the children were always fully clothed, childhood sleep-overs were not allowed, and, in some cases, the child was home schooled. The child was isolated from life's normal educational events that provided for a healthy understanding of sexuality. This environment created a vacuum of sexual information and experience. The vacuum imploded once he left the family environment. When he experienced sexual stimulation for the first time in his late teens or early twenties, it caused his system to go into overload, and, in turn, made sexual stimulation and orgasm exceptionally pleasurable and desirable. Compulsive repetition of the pleasurable experience turned into sex addiction.

Elijah's story

Elijah was raised in a very devout family. His parents believed children should be protected from the evils of society. Their five children were home schooled. They were not permitted to join scouting or sports activities. Elijah remembers childhood as a happy time. However, he did say he wished his father could have joined more family activities, but he didn't because of long hours of work.

Elijah said that during his childhood years, he didn't even know what sex meant. He remembers no discussion of bodily functions or human nature within the family environment. As a teenager, he did not date. The only exposure he had to girls was his two younger sisters. He remembers asking his mother what the word ". . ." meant that he saw written on the wall of a men's room. She dismissed his question by saying that he should not repeat bad words.

At age eighteen, Elijah was sent off to a small, parochial college. When his dorm mates found out he had never seen a *Playboy* magazine, they flooded him with pornography. Elijah said he devoured the magazines and began to masturbate daily. He felt he could not tell his parents about his sexual discovery. Elijah said, "As time went by my appetite for sexual material grew. I found that I could not stop, even when I wanted too." He finally talked to a clergy person about his sexual activity and was referred to a pastoral counselor.

Abbott's story

Abbott recalled that as a young child he was frequently ill. "My asthma prevented me from playing outdoors much of the year. My mother was fearful of childhood diseases carried by other children, and would not invite playmates into our home. I passed time by reading, viewing television, and playing video games. I became a loner."

In school, Abbott had just a couple friends. These friends were also interested in playing video games. Abbott said that he was afraid of girls and kept his distance. He said he remembers being teased by several girls because he was shy. He did not date during high school.

"During my late teen years, a new girl moved in next door. She had no drapes on her bedroom window. Each evening, I watched her from my bedroom window. I used binoculars to watch her undress. I found myself sexually stimulated and I learned to masturbate during my nightly viewing ritual."

At age nineteen, Abbott was arrested for peeping into windows in his neighborhood. As a form of alternative sentencing, he was required to participate in sex offender counseling.

Each of these men was sexually unaware during childhood. It was not until late in their development that they were exposed to sexual stimulation. For each, late exposure to sexual material was traumatic and formed the basis of their sexual addiction.

Model Two—Sexual Addiction Begins in Childhood

Most men who are sexually addicted as adults were exposed to a "catalytic event" during childhood. (Carnes, 1994) The "catalytic event" was age inappropriate exposure to sexual materials or behavior. Sexual addiction for most men begins in childhood—long before they understand what was happening. It happened before they were mentally mature enough to understand or able to exercise choices.

The following are several vignettes that include the characteristics generally found in the roots of sexually addicted men. They are recorded in detail to allow you to see how destructive age inappropriate exposure to sexual material and behavior can be. Each of the men in these vignettes did not realize they were becoming sexually addicted. They were introduced to sexuality at a time in their life when their human development did not allow them to make informed decisions. The vignettes show common themes about the beginning of sexual addiction. See if you can find them.

Jack's Story

From Jack's earliest memory, he recalls his mother tying him to a chair whenever he got in her way, which was often. He remembers his mother constantly yelling at him—telling him how he could do better. It was nearly impossible for him to satisfy his mother's expectations. She was a perfectionist. He was the older of two boys.

Jack's father was not around much. He often worked away from home for months at a time and when he was home, he did not have time for Jack. He had no memory of a pleasant conversation with his Dad. He does not remember his father ever taking time to teach him about sports or anything meaningful. What Jack remembers is his father's collection of pornographic magazines. Around age ten he found his father's collection. He recalls wondering why his father kept them. What impressed Jack most about the pornographic magazines were women with large breasts. When he stared at the pictures, he said he felt strange—what he now knows as arousal. His arousal feelings would turn to shame and guilt. His mother also had large breasts. He remembers, as a child, scanning the daily newspapers looking for images of women with large breasts. As a teenager, when he was home alone, he would go to his father's magazines and fantasize about having sex with one of the women pictured while he masturbated.

He has a very vivid memory of an encounter with his father. Around age twelve he remembers his enraged father stripping him naked in front of their home and beating him. Other children, including neighborhood girls, watched. Jack remembers a profound sense of humiliation and shame. Later he sought out one of the girls who had watched to engage in sexual activity with her. He felt hatred for her and his father.

As an adult, Jack thought it was all right to masturbate. All men do it, he thought. He continued to masturbate with the aid of pornographic pictures. As time went by, he sought human contact to stimulate himself. He began to visit massage parlors, often several times a week. He began to spend up to several thousand dollars a week on massage parlors. He also found much better pornographic material on the Internet. Jack estimates that at least 20 percent of his work week is spent thinking about sexual images or masturbating.

Ted's story

Ted remembers sexual activity as a young child. A neighbor boy seven years older first approached Ted when he was five years old. In time, the older boy taught Ted about oral sex. He has vivid memories of his first exposure to sexual activity. He remembers a tittilating feeling when the older boy touched him. He said he felt very confused but he liked the older boy's attention.

On the one hand Ted liked his new feelings but on the other he knew that what was happening was not right. The boys always had to hide in the garage and he was told not to tell anyone. He wondered why the older neighbor boy chose him—there were a lot of other boys in the neighborhood. Could there be something wrong with him? Did he cause it to happen? Was he bad? Why was he ashamed that it happened? He had wanted to tell his parents but thought that the older boy would have beaten him up if he told. He also thought his parents would punish him if they knew what he did.

While Ted was in his early grade-school years, several older neighborhood boys would get together for sex play (Ted was the youngest). A few years later Ted introduced several young neighborhood children to sex play. He said that his sex play with older boys continued into his early teenage years.

As a child and particularly as a teen, Ted did not have many friends. He was often teased because of his small stature. He made friends with a football player once but was devastated when his friend punched him in the face for petty reasons. Ted relates that he often cried himself to sleep. Today, he recognizes that he lived in depression. He felt isolated from his family and did not have much of a life. He did well academically because his parents put a premium on achieving good grades. However, no matter how hard he tried, it seemed that his parents thought he could do better. He was not close to either of them. His father was a military man and Ted was not a macho son. Ted's father had a continuing problem with alcohol. His mother was busy with her social life.

Ted did marry and he too joined the military. After he married, he thought that his wife used sex as a weapon to control him. When children came along, Ted absented himself from his family by accepting assignments that would take him away from them. When he was away, Ted used alcohol and masturbation to help him feel less lonely. He thought that his wife didn't love him.

Ted's thoughts turned to sex with men. He eventually made contact with others who considered sex among other married men a reasonable thing to do. Ted had an eighteen-month affair with a man who was about seven years older than he. Ted thought that this man was a potential companion and deep male friend—the male friendship he wanted all of his life. He subsequently learned that his male partner was only interested in sex.

Hank's story

Hank has early memories of sex. Both his parents would bring home sex partners, particularly when they were drunk. His father did nothing to conceal his sexual encounters from his children. While he knew well who his parents were supposed to be, he thought of his older brother and sister as his real parents.

Hank was angry, repulsed, and ashamed by his parent's behavior. He did not understand why some of his older brothers were not as repulsed as he was. As his brothers grew older, they brought home pornography and eventually sex partners. Hank wanted to escape his environment but did not know how. Eventually his father disappeared from the family and because of lack of money, his mother, brothers, and sisters moved to a government subsidized housing project. When Hank was about fourteen years old, an older woman, who lived on a floor above, asked him to help her. He did help her but it became clear that she wanted help with something else. She seduced Hank. The word got out and soon Hank was the new young stud in the project.

In his late teens, Hank vowed to escape. He moved to a town several hundred miles away. Unfortunately, Hank did not escape. He began to have affairs with several women simultaneously. He married one of the women with whom he had an affair. She wants him to give up all of his women. He is finding it very difficult to limit his sexual life to one woman.

Art's story

Art remembers being dressed up by his parents and hearing his relatives say how cute he looked. Family pictures show a boy of about three or four dressed in white tights and a frilly dress. He often wondered if his parents would have preferred a girl child.

Early in his life a grandmother cared for him. Art's mother worked and traveled frequently as part of her job. She would come home from business trips very tired and say she needed time to herself. He does not remember his mother as affectionate. In fact, he is sure that he was held and hugged but he cannot remember it happening. Art's father, like his mother, was not affectionate. He was busy with his business, which required most of his waking hours. In grade school the message he now remembers was: "We will love you even more if you get excellent grades in school." He strived hard to get excellent grades but it did not make much difference in how his parents treated him.

While in grade school and when his parents were not home, Art went to his mother's bedroom and dressed in her clothing. He particularly liked to dress in her white pantyhose. When he was around twelve years of age, his mother caught him dressed in her clothing. She immediately took him to his father for punishment. Both his parents shamed him by telling him how greatly he had disappointed them. He felt guilty for wanting to dress in his mother's clothing but did not know what to do about it. As a teen he became aroused when he dressed in female clothing and he looked forward to masturbating while viewing himself in the mirror.

Art thought he came from a loving family, but during therapy he began to question his thinking. Although he thinks he can talk to his parents, he still believes that their love is conditioned on how well he does in graduate school and how much money he earns.

As a young adult, Art periodically buys women's clothing and goes on a sex binge until he becomes disgusted with himself. He then trashes the clothing and tries to reform his ways. However, when he sees a woman dressed attractively, he forms a fantasy of himself wearing her clothes and masturbates while fantasizing.

Simon's story

Around age five, Simon was allowed to play unattended with neighborhood children up and down the street. Late one summer afternoon, he remembers being told by two older neighborhood girls that they wanted to play house with him. They took him to one of the girl's back yards and made a tent with blankets. Once inside the tent the girls undressed and touched him. They called it tickling. He felt very uncomfortable but liked the new feeling.

Time passed quickly and Simon realized that he was late for dinner. He was supposed to be home before the six o'clock fire whistle sounded. Upon hearing the whistle blow, he ran home. When he entered his home, his clothes were in disarray. His shirt was out, his pants were unbuttoned, and he was missing a sock. He felt frightened and was sure that he would be questioned about his state of undress. He really wanted to tell his mother what the girls had done with him. Instead his mother yelled at him for not being properly dressed. Why didn't his mother ask him why his clothes were in such disarray? Did she really know what he had been doing? He felt very confused.

Several weeks later, one of the older girls returned and took Simon into the woods across from where he lived. This time there were no blankets to hide under. A neighborhood child told Simon's father what was going on in the woods. Simon's father shamed him. Simon felt that he was a very bad boy.

As Simon grew, his interest in sex play with neighborhood children grew. He wondered what was wrong with him. Why did he seem to be the one interested in sex play?

As an adult, Simon married his school sweetheart. He now understands that he equated intimacy with sex. Sex was about the only real connection they had.

Simon felt isolated in his marriage and his wife's frequent criticism of him made him feel like the bad boy that he knew he had been all his life. Several years after his wedding an opportunity to tickle a young child presented itself. He found he could not resist. His feelings of guilt and shame were now compounded. In fact, he thought he could not be loved as bad as he thought he was. He began living in depression.

Jimmy's story

Jimmy was an affable boy around the age of ten. Both of Jimmy's parents were very involved in their professions. Jimmy's father was a workaholic lawyer. Jimmy's mother was a professor at a local college.

The family belonged to a prestigious country club with all the amenities of golf, tennis, swimming, and social events. Jimmy's parents worked during the day. During the summer they dropped Jimmy off at the country club on their way to work. Jimmy's schedule at the county club was filled with lessons. Early in the morning he had a golf lesson, followed by practice on the driving range. Early afternoon he had a tennis lesson. Often on the days when a tennis match did not follow his lesson, he would go swimming with other boys like himself.

Jimmy liked tennis because, as he understood later as an adult, Steve, the tennis pro, paid a lot of attention to him. Jimmy took to spending afternoon hours in the tennis shack with Steve. Steve taught him how to re-string a racket and other useful skills. One day while spending time with Steve, Jimmy said that he wanted to meet up with his friends and go swimming. However, that day Jimmy had forgotten to bring his swim trunks. Steve said he had a pair of swim trunks in the lost and found that probably would fit Jimmy. He suggested Jimmy try on the trunks at the tennis shack to see if they fit him. As he changed, Steve remarked that for a young boy he had a large penis. He asked Jimmy if he ever touched himself in order to make his penis hard. Steve asked him to show him how he did it. Jimmy felt uncomfortable but he did not want to disappoint his friend Steve, and complied with his request.

As the summer went on, Steve found more opportunities to initiate sexual stimulation with Jimmy. He introduced Jimmy to pornography. Jimmy liked the attention that Steve showed to him, and felt that perhaps their secret behavior was Steve's way of showing him how to be a man—at least that was what Steve said. Jimmy never shared his behavior with his parents. It seemed to him that a time when his parents were open to listening just never happened. Jimmy knew something was wrong with what was happening. He was confused over the conflict between the good feelings he experienced and the secrets Steve made him keep.

After the summer, Jimmy and Steve no longer saw each other. Steve moved to a warmer climate. Jimmy continued to masturbate whenever he felt he wanted to repeat the good feelings he first experienced with Steve. Jimmy began to masturbate more frequently.

Jimmy entered therapy in his early thirties to deal with compulsive masturbation and pornography. Jimmy was committed to shed his victimhood. His recovery journey took several years, and was successful.

Common Elements Found in the Roots of Sexual Addiction

Common elements in these vignettes

When you read these vignettes with which common elements did you identify? See if you can answer the following questions:

1. Approximately at what age or stage of their lives were the men introduced or witnessed sexual activity, material, or promiscuity?

_____

_____

_____

2. What type of relationship did the men have with their parents (close, neutral, distant, etc.)?

_____

_____

_____

3. How did they feel about their parents' involvement in their lives? What did the parents expect from them?

_____

_____

_____

4. Whom did they tell about their exposure to sex? Why?

_____

_____

_____

5. What did they think their parents' response would be if they told them about their exposure to sex?

_____

_____

_____

6. What feelings did the men express when they were introduced to sex? (See if you can find at least four expressions of feelings.)

_____

_____

_____

7. Was the introduction to sex a one-time happening? What happened as the men progressed through childhood and teen years?

_____

_____

_____

8. What happened to each man in his adulthood?

_____

_____

_____

9. Did any of the men repeat the sexual behavior they learned as children once they became adults? If yes, indicate how.

_____

_____

_____

10. Would you call any of the men sexually addicted as adults? Why?

_____

_____

_____

Common elements in your life

Let's now turn to you and look for these same characteristics in your life. Take the time to think about your childhood and answer the questions below. Likely you will think the effort is worthwhile. You may need additional space to answer some of these questions.

1. At what age or stage of life were you introduced to or witnessed sexual activity, material, or promiscuity? (Think carefully. For some men the exposure was not as clear as it was in the above cases. Don't be concerned if you cannot recall a childhood exposure. For some it will take some time and work to recall.)

_____

_____

_____

2. What type of relationship did you have with your parents (close, neutral, distant, etc.)?

    _____

    _____

    _____

3. What did you feel about your parents' involvement in your life? What did your parents expect from you?

    _____

    _____

    _____

4. Did you tell anyone about your first exposure to sex? Why?

    _____

    _____

    _____

5. What did you think your parents' response would be if you told them about your first exposure to sex?

    _____

    _____

    _____

6. What were your feelings when you were first introduced to sex? Did you feel an arousal when you were first exposed to sex? Did you feel shame or guilt when it was over? Were you confused? What did you do about your feelings?

    _____

    _____

    _____

7. Was your introduction to sex a one-time happening? What happened as you progressed through childhood and teen years?

_____

_____

_____

8. What happened to you in adulthood related to unwanted sexual behavior?

_____

_____

_____

9. Did you repeat the sexual behavior you learned as a child after you became an adult? How is your adult behavior similar to that which you were taught as a child?

_____

_____

_____

10. Would you call yourself sexually addicted? Why?

_____

_____

_____

Highlights of the Origin of Sexual Addiction

These vignettes and exercises focus on common family environments and early childhood exposure to age-inappropriate sexual stimulation that most sexually addicted adult men experienced during their childhood. Did you find your childhood experience similar to that of any of the men in the vignettes?

For some men, a life-changing event occurs later in life, which sets the stage for sexual addiction. Examples include rape or coming out of severe repression as a teen or adult. Late teenage or an adult onset of sexual addiction is less common than sexual addiction with roots in childhood.

Paul Becker, LPC

It is now time to give a brief summary of the origin of sexual addiction. There may be other elements. We will only explore those that research has proven to apply to large numbers of sexually addicted men. It is impossible to say that this or any other model applies to all men who deal with unwanted sexual behavior. However, the prevalence is high enough to allow the following generalizations.

When presenting highlights of the origin of sexual addiction, I will not go into great detail. In Appendix B, you will find scholarly research references. My intent here is not to make you a trained, fully informed clinical practitioner. It is to help you decide if you have a sexual addiction problem and to share ideas of where you may wish to go next.

In his book, *Contrary to Love*, Carnes (1994), explores the elements of addiction in far greater detail. If you choose to do something about your unwanted sexual behavior, read as many of Patrick Carnes' books as you can during your journey through recovery. See Appendix B for a list of his works. He and his associates are the premier experts in healing of sexual addiction.

Age-inappropriate exposure to sexual behavior or material

A young child cannot be exposed to sexual behavior or material without consequences. A child does not have the life experiences to put such an event into perspective. Our sexuality begins very early in life and nature intends it to evolve as we age. It is very normal for a young child to touch his genitals. It is not normal for a person other than a loving care giver to touch a child. A child instinctively knows the difference.

A child also instinctively knows that pornographic material is not part of his normal environment. Such exposure is traumatic to a child. For many, it is a trauma that they will remember for the rest of their lives. If parents do not normalize the event (explain and put it into perspective for the child) it may be a beginning factor which will lead to sexual addiction later in life.

Family environment and structure

Most sexually addicted men come from a family environment that did not meet their childhood needs for affection or emotional support. Often children who live in dysfunctional families feel a sense of abandonment by their parents. The parents simply were not there for the child in a way that led to feelings of self-confidence and love. The child felt isolated from his parents and his siblings.

The family was usually either rigid or chaotic. If the family was rigid, the child thought that he had to measure up to his parents' expectations of him or he may have concluded that he was not a worthy human being. Family rules were conveyed explicitly, often by yelling, critical nagging, or body language. Body language in a rigid family may include the deep sigh, a frown, abruptly disconnected conversation, or the look that could kill. In either mode, the child receives the message that he is deficient. A rigid family is often performance-based. That is, for the child to be loved, he has to perform. Getting good grades, doing well in sports, and having a physically fit body are some examples of conditional love. The child frequently thinks that it is not possible for him to perform in the way his parents require. The adage, "Children are to be seen and not heard," is characteristic of a rigid family. The family is run by a system of rules. Punishment for not abiding the rules of behavior is often accompanied by parental scorn.

In his book, *Facing the Shadow*, Carnes (2010) says:

> Sex addicts also tend to come from rigid, authoritarian families. These are families in which all issues and problems are black and white. Little is negotiable and there is only one way to do things. Success in the family means doing what the parents want to such an extent that children give up being whom they are. Normal child development does not happen. By the time children enter adolescence, they have few options. One is to become rebellious. The other is to develop a secret life about which the family knows nothing. Both positions distort reality. Both result in a distrust of authority and a poor sense of self.

> If the family's rigidity is also sex negative (that is, children are taught that sex is dirty, sinful, bad, or nasty), sex becomes exaggerated or hidden. Worse yet, the forbidden can become the object of obsession. Or all of the above may happen. The worst-case scenario happens when the child finds out that parents are not living up to their sexual standards. For example, if the parents preach against sexual promiscuity but one or both chronically have affairs, this teaches the acceptability of sexual duplicity. The norm is to deceive others and to pretend that what is true is not true.

The chaotic family is on the opposite end of the spectrum. A child in a chaotic family thinks he has no thoughts that are his own. His parents are always penetrating the boundaries of his world. The child has no space he can call his own. In a chaotic situation the family name is of paramount importance. It is the job of all family members to look good to the neighbors. If a member of the family fails, it was the job of the family to close ranks and protect the wounded member.

In both a rigid and a chaotic family, the child ends up feeling the same. He is not loved for whom he is as a human being. Such children feel isolated and seek other avenues to express themselves. For some it becomes sex, even though sex is often considered bad or dirty and is rarely talked about.

When a child feels isolated and detached from his parents, he is unable to go to them with confidence that they will love him when something bad has happened. For most young children who are exposed to age-inappropriate behavior or material, instinct tells them that something bad has happened. Their fear of parental discovery discourages them from seeking the very healing that comes from parental intervention.

This is the very time that a child needs his parents most. It is critical that parents are called upon to explain to the child that his exposure to age-inappropriate behavior or material was not his fault, and as a child, he could not be responsible. Parental guidance is needed to explain that the normal body reaction to sexual touch or material—arousal—is not bad. It is normal at the proper time and circumstances. A traumatized child needs to know that he is loved unconditionally and that this bad event does not change his parents' love.

When a child believes he cannot trust his parents to love him at the time of exposure to age-inappropriate behavior or material, he withdraws into himself and becomes even more isolated. He now has a huge troubling secret that he believes he cannot share. Many children even begin to blame themselves for the event, when all the logical signs point elsewhere. The child is often permanently damaged.

Arousal

Arousal is the normal consequence of sexual stimulation—it is how God made us. Babies engage in self-stimulation, which is a normal process of self-discovery and learning the response to touch. But for a child who is introduced to sexual material or sex acts, the arousal is out of the norm. A child instinctively knows what normal stimulation is and realizes that the arousal he is experiencing is abnormal.

One of the reasons is intensity. When a child is first stimulated by sexual material or through the acts of another person, the intensity of the arousal is greater than normal self-stimulation. The child feels flooded with new feelings. For the first time the brain is encoding the intensity of the feelings and that encoding may remain for a lifetime. Do you remember the first time that you were stimulated by sexual material or through the acts of another person?

Do you remember the who, what, when, where? Why do you remember that experience with such clarity and not what you had for dinner on your birthday that year—another special occasion? Because the event was encoded in your brain, it was one of the defining moments of your life.

While you may have felt other emotions, your brain remembers the chemical flow, the arousal feelings. Drug addicts who use cocaine tell researchers that the first high on cocaine is the best they have ever experienced. Many report that their continued use is an attempt to recreate the first high. Likewise, without realizing it, many sexually addicted men try to recreate their first experience. For many, the sexual activity in which they engage as an adult has similar characteristics to sexual stimulus and arousal experienced in early childhood. For example, a child introduced to pornography may continue to be drawn to pornography as an adult. A child who is sexually abused is more likely to abuse other children in adulthood than a person who was not abused as a child.

Why do some children who are exposed to unwanted sexual material or acts not go on to have difficulty with adult sexual addiction? The relationship between the child and parent makes the difference. When a child feels comfortable telling a parent what has happened, and a parent is skilled in helping the child to understand that the child was not responsible for what happened, reassuring him that arousal is a normal consequence of stimulation, the child will likely not be as affected as a child who is unable to seek normalization from a parent. The relationship between the child and parent is critical in defusing the intensity of the event.

Feelings of shame, guilt, and depression

Shame and guilt are not the same. A man feels guilty when he knows he has done something wrong. Feelings of guilt can lead a man to change his behavior. Feelings of guilt emanate from his conscience talking to him. A shamed man feels something is wrong with him. John Bradshaw (1988) states, "Guilt says I've made a mistake; shame says I am a mistake. Guilt says what I did was not good; shame says I am no good. The difference makes a profound difference."

Bradshaw (1988) goes on to say:

> Shame with its accompanying loneliness and psychic numbness fuels our compulsive/addictive lifestyle. Shame is like a hole in the cup of our soul. Since the child in the adult has insatiable needs, the cup cannot be filled . . . . No matter how many times we fill the cup—the hole remains.

> Shame fuels compulsivity, and compulsivity is the black plague of our time. We are driven. We want more money, more sex, more food, more booze, more drugs, more adrenalin rush, more entertainment, more possessions, more ecstasy. Like an unending pregnancy, we never reach fruition.

Shame is a destructive feeling. It contributes to a sense of sadness and to depressed moods. To feel better, acting out sexually is a form of self-medication. Unfortunately the good feeling of an orgasm is quickly followed by shame and the cycle begins again. Addiction and obsessive disorders are symptoms of being abandoned and shamed in childhood, according to Bradshaw (1988).

When a child is first sexually aroused by age-inappropriate behavior or material, he knows that his feelings are different. He knows that what has happened generally occurred in a secretive environment. He may be told not to tell. He may know it was wrong. He may feel guilt but, more importantly, the mind of a child is programmed to feel that he is bad, that something is terribly wrong with him. A child's sense of shame is ignited by age-inappropriate sexual events. So much so that the feeling of shame, "I am defective," often stays with him for many years to come.

It is normal for a child to think he is at fault when something bad happens. For example, when the parents divorce, it is common for therapist to hear the child say, "If only I had been a better boy, Mom and Dad would not have separated." The same cross-wired thinking occurs here. When victimized by age-inappropriate behavior or material, the child frequently assumes he is at fault.

Paul Becker, LPC

John Bradshaw (1988) says:

> For example, if the parents are abusive and hurt the child through physical, sexual, emotional or mental pain, *the child will assume the blame, make himself bad, in order to keep the all-powerful protection against the terrors of night.* For a child at this stage to realize the inadequacies of parents would produce unbearable anxiety.

So the future sexually addicted person is isolated from his parents and feels at fault by the sexual experience. It is an easy jump to see that the child begins to live in some level of depression. Depression often follows the victim into adulthood.

For many men, the level of depression is not full-blown but low-grade. Low-grade differs from full depression only to the degree of the impact on one's daily functioning. For example, a fully depressed man may be unable to sleep properly, eat, or concentrate on the business at hand. Conversely, a man suffering low-grade depression functions each day but thinks he is missing the joys of life, feels tired much of the time, and finds the act of living a burden. Such a person wakes up and says "Oh, good God, not another day," instead of "Good God, thanks for another day." This state of malaise goes on for years. It becomes painful and the prospect of escape through sex is inviting. Sex becomes a way of self-medicating the pain of life. Depression, as a causal factor or consequence of sexual addiction, is addressed in Chapter 6.

Learned model in childhood that is repeated in adulthood

Do you ever look in the mirror and see your father? Do you see yourself repeating behaviors you once witnessed as a child? Behavior taught in childhood is often repeated in adulthood, even behavior that is despised by the child. So too, unwanted sexual behavior from childhood becomes unwanted sexual behavior in adulthood. Early childhood attachment to pornography is often repeated in adulthood. Abused children may abuse as adults. Children exposed to parental adulterous affairs may do likewise as adults. In fact, a high percent of sexually addicted men come from families where other addictions were present. If you are looking for the link to the type of unwanted sexual behavior that is giving you a problem today, look back into your childhood. You are likely to find the trail.

Richard's story

Every time Richard brought home a report card his father would go on at great length about the C that could be turned into a B, and the B that needed to be an A. His father never addressed the improvements that were made from the last report card, only the grades that needed improvement. It was a no win game, Richard concluded. This same scenario was repeated each report period through college. In college, Richard once received all A's, except for one B. His father focused on the B. In graduate school, Richard earned an all A semester. His father looked at the transcript, put it down, and walked away without saying a word.

Many years later Richard talked to his adult son, Leo, about memories of growing up. Leo said he had many good memories but he really did not like how his father (Richard) always focused on what could be improved in school rather than what Leo had achieved. Richard was stunned. He realized that he had repeated his father's behavior—the behavior that had hurt him deeply. How did that happen?

Richard's father sent him messages to the effect, "There is always room for improvement" and "A child needs to be encouraged to do better." These messages were packed away in Richard's adult bags. He hadn't unpacked his baggage from his childhood. Unless Leo unpacks his baggage from Richard, he is likely to pass the same messages, the same baggage, onto his children. Behavior, messages, and attitudes tend to be passed down from one generation to the next unless someone in the chain makes the effort to end the cycle. Is it time for you to be that person before you pass your addiction onto your children?

Are you now able to answer the question, "Why me?"

Pleasure that is obtained by unreasonable and unsuitable cost, must always end in pain

Samuel Johnson

Chapter Three

Why Can't I Just Stop?

Chances are that you have promised yourself many times that you will stop your unwanted sexual behavior. Perhaps you have stopped for short periods of time, but invariably you give in to sexual urges and return to old habits of acting out. In this chapter we will discuss a number of factors that keep sexually addicted men attached to their unwanted sexual behavior.

Brain Indoctrination

Habit

Multi tasking has become a byword in our society. The news media show clips of people talking on cell phones while driving, eating while driving, and even reading the newspaper or a book while driving. Why do people think they can do at least two things at once? Multi tasking drivers believe that their driving skill has become so indoctrinated into their brains that they no longer need to think about responses to road situations.

Sexual acting out is not like driving a car on the interstate but the call to act out has been similarly indoctrinated into the brain. Perhaps an applicable word is habit. People rely on habit-based skills to drive vehicles, and sex addicts repeat unwanted behavior partially out of habit. Habits are usually formed over many years. As we discovered in the last chapter, sexually acting out often begins during youth and is brought forward into adulthood.

The habit of acting out begins to define the personality. The adult sex addict begins to see life through the prism of sex. Much of his life takes on a sexual orientation. For example, when an addict sees a woman, man, or (sadly) children, he first surveys the body parts to see if they match his internal concept of what is sexually stimulating. Rarely does he focus on the woman's eyes or face first; he doesn't see a whole woman but focuses on body parts as objects. The habit of checking out breasts, legs, buttocks, etc., becomes so ingrained that it defines how he views humanity. People are not people to him but objects for sexual gratification. So too, when an addicted man picks up a book, magazine, or newspaper, his first instinct is not for the intellectual content of the publication but to look for images that may sexually stimulate his mind. Sex becomes his number one focus and his number one need.

Sexual fantasies

Many sexually addicted men live for exciting sexual fantasies. A man will see an attractive woman, store the images in his brain and then construct a fantasy of sexual activity with that person. Sexual fantasies are part of the brain's indoctrination since they serve as a launching platform for acting out. Looking for new and exciting sexual fantasies becomes a way of life and occupies much of the sex addict's time. Some sex addicts become so attached to the process they can't go to sleep without their favorite fantasy. While sexual fantasies are most often used to arouse, they are also used to calm stress. Sexual fantasies produce a sense of euphoria. They medicate life's pain. Sexual fantasies are a large part of the addiction and are very difficult to let go once they have become habitual.

An abused person can also use sexual fantasies as a defense mechanism. Often when a child is traumatized by sexual abuse, the mind of the abused child dissociates from reality. When the mind dissociates, it compartmentalizes what is happening in the present time and focuses on a mental sequence of another time and place or a fantasy or daydream absent of the pain of the present moment. The child uses dissociation to survive the trauma of abuse. Later in life the dissociation skill is again put to use in the form of a pleasurable sexual fantasy to deal with the pain of life.

Altering the brain

The brain is the center of addiction. The brain determines what is pleasurable and what is not. It also determines a degree of pleasure or pain. Pleasure from normal activities, reading a book, eating an ice cream cone, taking a walk, going to a movie, does not lead to addiction. Each of these activities, while pleasurable, is not likely to program the brain so that one compulsively seeks to repeat the behavior. However, the pleasure from sexual activity, as intended by nature, is highly enjoyable. It is one way that nature helps the human race to perpetuate itself. During sexual activity, the brain's chemicals tell it, "That was so pleasurable; I would like to do it again." The brain remembers that message and encourages the addict to repeat the sexual activity to generate pleasurable feelings. When this happens over and over, particularly when it begins in youth, the brain's neurotransmitters become very sensitive to the need for sexual stimulation. The brain becomes patterned and repeatedly calls for renewed flow of chemical activity that the brain finds so pleasurable. The brain has been altered. It now considers repetitive sexual stimulation normal.

When orgasm occurs, the brain is charged with endorphins. It records the experience as a euphoric moment. Obviously, the brain tells its component part, "Wow, that was fun." Some runners talk about a runner's high, an experience they like to repeat. An orgasm causes a significant "rush," an experience men like to repeat. Did you ever wonder why the feeling during an orgasm doesn't last? The simplistic answer is that when endorphins are used up, so is the euphoric feeling. This explains why a man no longer feels romantic after he has achieved a climax. The normal state of the brain is altered during the build up and orgasm.

Feelings of low mood and even pain are overridden by the chemical flow of endorphins. It is the combination of the reduction in pain and the feeling of euphoria that makes acting out sexually such a powerful experience—one that becomes compulsive for the addict.

Association of systems

Sexual activity does not occur in a vacuum. It takes place at locations and at selective times. The sexual act is associated with other people, objects (clothing, sex toys, etc.), moods, smells, and, at times, taste. These related systems remind the brain that pleasure is associated with the place, time, a person, smell, taste, etc. For example, an associated system for an alcoholic may be his neighborhood bar and his drinking friends. The alcoholic may tell himself that he is just going for an evening walk. However, if he walks anywhere near his favorite bar or encounters any of his drinking friends, his brain triggers an associative response, and his next drink is very near. Once the associative systems kick in, the alcoholic's power to resist is vastly reduced.

Likewise, the sex addict has associated systems that lure him back to unwanted sexual activity. For example, the man who is addicted to Internet pornography will convince himself time and again he is only going online to check e-mail. However, his brain knows by past experience that the act of turning on the computer is the first step toward sexual pleasure. Once the e-mail is checked, the addict may tell himself he just needs to check some other sites for whatever reason. The process continues until the addict finds a link that takes him down the road to pornography and acting out. Carnes (1994) calls this ritualization. A discussion of the acting out ritual follows later in this chapter.

A sexually addicted man has difficulty changing his lifestyle so that associative trigger systems are no longer part of his life. Such a lifestyle change can be difficult and may have high-priced consequences. If a man goes to the TV each evening in search of provocative images or scenes as a prelude to masturbation, giving away the TV may seem an unacceptable price. Placing filter software on a computer may affect legitimate as well as pornographic sites. The inability to link to legitimate sites is often used as an excuse not to block pornographic sites.

Isolation

Hiding behind the mask

Let's face it, you are not likely to walk up to each new person you meet and say, "Hi I'm John, I masturbate every chance I get." In fact, chances are you will label your problem by socially acceptable terms like stress, anxiety, depression, anger, not being loved, marriage problems—anything but "unwanted sexual behavior." Do you think you have a need to hide behind a mask of respectability? Do you have a very hard time admitting to yourself that you can't control your sexual activity, even though you have tried many times? Does your heart say to you, "If I admit to my wife or friends that my unwanted sexual activity has taken hold of my life, they may reject or abandon me?" Are you afraid that your shameful secret will get out and your world may collapse?

Are you terrified that others will think what you already think, that "I am a bad person?" Stop there—You are not bad. Your behavior may be undesirable, but God does not make bad people. The concept of feeling one's self as bad is a childlike response that may come from messages sent by your parents in childhood. The conclusion, "I am bad," is dead wrong. However, feeling bad has led you to isolation and to hide behind the mask of respectability.

What's more, your fears of being judged as "bad" may be overblown. The percentage of men who deal with unwanted sexual behavior sometime during their lives is high, some experts think close to half. The Internet produces men who are dealing with sexual acting out at a very high rate. You may be pleasantly surprised that many will applaud your recognition of your sexual addiction because you have accepted responsibility to do something about it. Many lack your courage. Coming out of isolation is key to recovery and will be addressed in Chapter 9.

Loneliness to isolation

Isolation is a consequence, of growing up in a family structure in which the child is not valued just for being himself. The child has learned well to withdraw so as not to subject himself to humiliation or verbal abuse. The child learned when he shared himself, his needs, feelings, dreams, and nonconforming thoughts he was ridiculed or even worse ignored. The survival mode quickly became isolation. Perhaps there are sexually addicted people who are not isolated, but they are few and far between. The price of isolation is loneliness. Since the isolated child did not learn normal socialization skills, the consequences of childhood isolation spill over into adulthood. Interestingly, isolated people are even isolated after they marry.

Carnes (2010) notes the lack of intimacy as a causal factor for loneliness:

> Most sex addicts, however, come from families in which members are "disengaged" from one another—there is little sharing or intimacy. Children develop few skills about sharing, being vulnerable, or risking anything about themselves. As a result, they learn to trust no one but themselves in such families. The further result is that self-delusion is then hard to break, and secrets become more potent than reality. The worst effect is that the children are unable to ask for help.

Codependency

Isolated men, quite unconsciously, often seek and find a marriage partner who has similar characteristics or deficiencies as their mothers. If a man's mother was condescending and critical, his partner will be, too. If his mother found it difficult to show affection, his partner will also find it difficult.

Codependency is found in many marriages where the male is sexually addicted. Chapter 5 is devoted to a full discussion of the role codependency may play in your marriage.

Sex to medicate pain

Let's agree, sex feels good while it lasts. If one is in a constructive marriage relationship, sex is one form of glue that helps the married couple stay together. While sex will rarely sustain a marriage all by itself, it is a blessing to be enjoyed as one would a delightful piece of fruit. Sex in this context also helps the couple to deal with the annoying side of life's little problems—dented fender, burnt steak, toilet seat left up, etc.

When a partner is isolated and the marriage does not provide the loving environment an addict needs, or if he is single with few meaningful relationships, acting out helps the addict deal with life's pain. However, for the addict, sex changes from a fruit to medication. It becomes the bandage strip that comes off in short order. Acting out sexually then is a can of plastic bandage strips. The problem is that the bandages never act to heal—they just temporarily cover up life's difficulties and pain.

Sexual abuse as a child

As stated earlier, Carnes (1992) found that 81 percent of addicts he surveyed remember being abused sexually in some way as a child. When a child is introduced to age-inappropriate sexual activity, material, or stimulation and he is a product of family in which normal emotional nourishment is not available to the child, the likelihood that he, in time, will become sexually addicted is very high.

In a dysfunctional family the child learns that parental love is conditional. So much so that he learns he has to take care of his own emotional needs to survive. The child becomes isolated and finds that sexual activity provides the good feeling he would otherwise look to receive from his parents, siblings, friends, or other healthy activities.

The combination of an inappropriate sexual stimulus at a young age and dysfunctional family life is a formula for addiction.

Sex Addiction Cycle

Men who deal with unwanted sexual behavior find themselves repeating time and again a cycle of thinking and events called a "sex addiction cycle." It is akin to the proverbial donkey being locked to the wine press. He goes round and round, even when he would rather not.

In *Contrary to Love*, (1994) Carnes describes the sex addiction cycle. This section is an adaptation of his concept.

One of the principal characteristics of addiction is that the act is repetitive to the point in which the addict becomes powerless to change the outcome. Each time he goes through the acting out process he completes a cycle. In short, there is a beginning thought process, a build up, the act, the let down (guilt, grief, pledges to do better, and self-justification), and a return to the beginning.

Below are sequential steps or phases sexually addicted men experience. Within each phase the addict will engage in thinking described in one or more of the subtitles under each phase. The time an addict takes to repeat the cycle can vary from minutes to months.

Initial Phase—Life Condition

Victim posture. In this belief system, I am a victim in this world and not responsible for my behavior. In a new situation, I look for ways I will be hurt. I may not even know that I look to be a victim. I have poor boundaries—people take advantage of me.

Low-grade depression. Life for me is an existence; I often think life is passing me by. Except when acting out, I am rarely happy and I never feel joy.

Anticipated rejection. I create situations in which someone else can reject me. I hold people at a distance. I can't let people know my real self—I know they will not love me.

Social isolation. I live behind a mask of respectability but underneath my mask is my real self. I simply cannot let anyone in. If I did, they would see that I am really a bad person. I have few or no real friends. No one really knows who I am.

Emotional isolation. I am neither in touch with my own feelings nor with other people's feelings. I don't understand that I hurt others. I don't understand my own feelings. For me, intimacy means sex.

Mood change. I perceive even small events as being negative. When my mood goes negative, acting out follows.

Phase Two—Reaction to Life Condition

Escapism. Living life is just too boring or life is just one painful experience after another. I need to find ways of relieving my bad feelings.

Need-fulfilling fantasy. I don't know how to cope. Thus, I daydream of a better life. I use fantasy to get temporary relief.

Sexual fantasy. I use sexual fantasies or visual sexual stimulation to escape my pain. My next act is often the subject of my fantasies and my sexual thinking. My fantasy is my best friend—we see each other a lot.

Sexual materials. I maintain a well-used collection of pornographic magazines and movies, web sites, and sex toys. Whenever I feel lonely, tired, or angry, my stash is nearby to raise my mood.

Phase Three—Acting out

Acting out ritual. I mentally begin a ritual that leads to acting out. At times I play games with myself. For examples, I tell myself I will just go a little way but not all the way—but then I go all the way. I go to the Internet to check mail and end up at a porn site.

Phase Four—Reconciliation

Transitory guilt. I feel sorry and ashamed of myself. I fear being caught. My focus is on what is going to happen to me. I am unaware of how I hurt my family. My feeling of guilt is short-lived.

Reconstruction. I present outwardly that I am a good guy. I seek forgiveness at church. I am never going to do it again. I am going to make it right. I conceal my act.

Mistaken beliefs. I didn't hurt anybody. I deserve some pleasure in life. Sex is my most important need. I act out sexually even when I don't want to.

Thinking errors. I can control it if I want to. I don't need any help. What do they know about my problem?

Once completed, the addict returns to the initial phase and begins the cycle anew.

Acting Out Ritual

Every addict repeats a ritual (phase three) before acting out. According to Carnes (1994):

> The ritual seems magically to bring order out of chaos. Think of it as a dance—certain steps, certain sounds, ceremony, rhythm, special artifacts—which can be very elaborate but have one purpose: to put addicts into another world so they can escape the conditions of real life over which they think they have no control. Fantasy is compounded by delusion at this point, for the mood-altered state is a "world" in which the addicts no longer care about control in the same way. Sexual obsession is pursued to its peak regardless of risk, harm, or other consequences. There is only one kind of control that matters now—control of sexual pleasure. Once they start dancing, they rarely, if ever, can stop on their own.

Rituals are often connected to places, things, or activities. For example, Mason knew the location of all the massage parlors in his city. He would cruise the neighborhoods nearby, tell himself he was not going near a massage parlor, but found himself repeatedly parking nearby. For others, the rituals may include visiting parks, swimming pools, shopping malls, restrooms, movie theaters, porn shops, peep shows, or other locations that are part of the pattern used by the addict to set the stage for acting out. The TV remote is a curse for many men. Channel flipping might be compared to having a gun with one round in the chamber. Sooner or later a channel will provide the visual stimulation needed to activate the lust pattern.

Men are usually not cognizant of the consistency of their ritualization patterns until they are asked to record the events that lead to an orgasm. They are even more surprised to discover their ritual often begins long before they take any action. Initial steps in the ritual may begin with feelings of Hunger, Anger, Loneliness, and Tiredness, often referred to by the acronym HALT. Since addicted men frequently live in a state of low-grade depression, the feeling of being down may trigger a need to alter their mood and thus their ritual.

Sexually addicted men have one or more acting out rituals. Once the addict has passed through the initial steps of his ritual, he hits a slippery slope. Picture a ski slope. While at the bottom of the slope, he still has choices. The mind of the addict doesn't correlate riding the chair lift with acting out, so he stands in line and rides to the top of the slope. While standing at the top, he can convince himself that a leisurely ride will not result in acting out, but he must be careful not to gain too much speed or to hit a patch of ice that will render him out of control. While cruising through long, sweeping turns, feeling comfortable, the mind of the addict wants to go a little faster and even faster after that. Suddenly the addict is barreling down the slippery slope toward certain sexual acting out and he doesn't understand why. The mind of the addict isn't willing to consider all the decisions that brought him to the speed and direction he is currently taking. Instead, he blames a patch of ice or the slope itself. The slippery slope of his addiction begins when he sees the chair lift, not when his speed and direction no longer allow him to stop.

Greg's story

Greg longed for the touch of a female. Massage parlors that specialized in oral sex or masturbation was Greg's sexual life line. From Greg's point of view, the stress of his high paying job justified a means to seek relief from his charged-up daily life. For him, the answer was to go to a massage parlor each Friday afternoon.

Greg began to realize massage parlors did not make him happy. He constantly looked for a better experience time and again, but he was never satisfied. Through the help of his counselor he began to record his acting out rituals. Together they looked for the event or change in mood that began his descent to acting out. They called Greg's descent his slippery slope. Greg learned he could stop the mental processing at an initial stage. Once he was past the initial stages of his descent, he could no longer stop. He was on the slippery slope.

Greg outlined his acting out ritual in the following steps:

- During the week Greg's mind would process past trips to one or more massage parlors. He would think about the woman with the best technique—the woman who satisfied him the most. Thinking about past experiences kept his sexual tension high during the week.

- Greg constantly looked for someone who could excite him more. He liked to try out new parlors in search of what he called the Holy Grail. He liked to engage in fantasies of what he called the perfect touch.

- Wednesday's local newspaper contained ads for massage parlors. Greg waited in anticipation of reading it.

- When a new ad appeared, Greg would call to set up an appointment. He often found new ads.

- Friday mornings were times of very high sexual energy. At times Greg would masturbate in his office so that the afternoon's experience would last longer.

- Greg drove his older car to work on Fridays. He thought he was less likely to be identified in his Honda Accord than in his BMW.

- Greg cleared his calendar for Friday afternoons so that he could leave the office by 3:00 P.M.

- When Greg got into his car Friday afternoon, he occasionally would have second thoughts like, "Maybe I can skip it today." He would tell himself that he would just go to Starbucks for a coffee. Invariably, he found himself driving through the neighborhood of the massage parlor, even when he told himself that he was going to Starbucks.

- Greg went to a massage parlor just about every Friday afternoon. He found he could no longer stop himself.

Greg thought his slippery slope began when he mentally processed past encounters. Although this step was critical to beginning his descent, Greg's mental processing was in the riding the chair lift phase. He needed to examine why he stood in the chair lift line in the first place.

The issue Greg needed to address was his stress. Unless he managed his stress in a constructive way, he would likely return to his entitlement logic, "I need this to come down from my charged-up daily life."

Acting out rituals are preprogrammed series of events or thoughts that the addict steps through before engaging in sexual activity. The addict needs to get in touch with his own acting out ritual and identify at what point he can interdict the ritual to change the sexual response.

Environmental Temptation

At times life in the United States is a paradox. We are horrified at sexual crime and rightly so. Yet, sex is the prime motivator behind much of our advertising. We sell pornographic magazines out in the open (Playboy, Hustler, etc.). We allow porn sites to dominate the Internet. Then we are shocked to learn that Joe is dealing with sexual addiction. Joe is attracted to porn for many reasons, and we have made it easy for him to nourish his addiction. Sexual stimulation is everywhere—advertising, regular TV programming, billboards, beach, sports cheerleaders, MTV, and on and on. Environmental temptation is a serious problem for many.

Are You Discouraged?

Perhaps after reading this chapter, you are discouraged. Perhaps you thought it would be relatively easy to rid yourself of unwanted sexual behavior. Unfortunately, for most men the journey takes a lifetime. The good news is that many men have chosen to begin the journey. In Chapter 7 we talk about hope—the first ingredient to recovery.

What is the greatest problem? Some believe that giving up or despair is the ultimate pitfall. When one gives up and continues in their sex addictive behavior, then they are accepting "no hope" as their answer. If you fall from your horse named "sobriety" the first subsequent action for you is to get back up and continue your journey. Many men are tempted to act out again once they have fallen and justify themselves through all sorts of "stinking thinking." Continuing to lie on the ground and continue to act out is a defeatism attitude. Look at the positive. For example, if you had two weeks of sobriety and succumbed to the urge to act out, it is much more productive to say, "I had a month of sobriety, with a short interruption at week two. After a month or two the fall at week two no longer matters. What matters is that you are continuing to move forward on your recovery journey.

**Self-respect is the root of discipline; the sense of dignity grows
with the ability to say no to oneself.**

Abraham J. Heschel

**Treat your mind like a bad neighborhood—
don't go there alone.**

Source Unknown

Chapter Four

Pornography

Pornography is the millstone around the neck of a sexually addicted man. Perhaps the number one reason sexually addicted men enter therapy is to deal with addiction to pornography. Most have been caught viewing pornography online by their wife, significant other, or employer.

Men crave a return to the secrecy of sexual stimulation that occurred during childhood. They mistakenly believe they can go online and enjoy their own secret world of sexual stimulation and never get caught. A pattern repeated by many men is to stay up late—after their wives have gone to sleep—and search the Internet for sexually stimulating images.

Bart's story

Bart believed viewing online pornography did not affect his marriage. Bart was an upwardly mobile young executive and often took work home. He had an agreement with his wife that he would not do office work while she and the children were awake. After Bart's wife retired for the evening, Bart went online. He would spend an hour or two attending to office work, but then succumbed to the temptation to view pornographic material. He felt he deserved to reward himself, for he was an outstanding breadwinner and his wife did not seem to need sexual activity as much as he did. He looked forward to viewing pornography and subsequent masturbation.

His wife was a sound sleeper and never disturbed his late night sessions on the computer. That was, until one night when she walked in on him, and saw what

48

she called "sick" images on his computer. Not only did she see the images on his computer, but he was in the process of masturbating when she walked in.

Bart's wife, like any normal wife, was traumatized by her husband's behavior. She told him that unless he got help, their relationship was likely over. Now Bart was devastated. Bart entered therapy, but found the road back to sexual sobriety more difficult than he expected. After a year of therapy, Bart continued to go three times a week to a Twelve Step program to keep himself straight. He also found that an exercise program helped him maintain a better mental disposition. Having been discovered, Bart said, was initially the worst thing that could have happened to him. He now realizes it was the opportunity for life changing choices, and a far better relationship with his wife.

Men also go online from their computers at work and believe they will not get caught.

Bill's story

Bill was an IT guy who believed he could defeat any filter or tracking tools used by his employer. His employer was a State government. However, it was not the controls that his employer put on the system that caused Bill to lose his "dream" position. One Friday afternoon he was called into his supervisor's office and told to pack up his things. He was no longer an employee. His supervisor explained to him that a female coworker filed a sexual harassment complaint after she observed pornographic images on Bill's computer as she passed by his work cubicle. Bill was devastated. His wife was outraged. The family was in crisis. A major problem faced by the family was paying for the medical care of their disabled son. Bill was able to obtain freelance work to barely keep the family afloat. Bill, and his family paid a high price for the lure of pornographic images.

Art's story

Art's employer made it clear that anyone caught viewing pornography at the work site would be fired. Art was a highly specialized engineer, and thought, no matter what he did, he would never be fired. His company needed his expertise. Art's pattern of behavior was to view online pornography after his coworkers left for the day. He got caught, and was told by his boss that he had one more chance. He failed to take stock of the warning. He was subsequently fired for his activity on a company computer. Art entered therapy to try to convince his boss he was serious about changing his behavior. Art learned it was not his boss whom he needed to satisfy, but himself. He made good progress in therapy and is employed by another company.

Definition of pornography

Defining pornography for universal acceptance is nearly impossible. You may wish to go online to find a definition that meets your standards. For the purposes of this book we use an oversimplified definition.

Pornography is any sexually stimulating material or language that is used by a sexually addicted person to foster sexual stimulation.

While sexually stimulating material may be used by married couples, even such use falls within our definition if the focus of the sexually addicted man is more on the stimulating images than on his wife. Some find it hard to believe that pornography of any type is healthy within the marriage. Why does a man or a woman need external materials to facilitate sexual arousal? In such cases, other issues are at work which precludes marital intimacy. They need to be addressed.

The simplistic approach toward a definition means any material a man uses to foster sexual stimulation is pornography for him. As indicated earlier, pornography may or may not be the type found at an adult bookstore. One man found lingerie ads in newspapers and catalogs to be his form of pornography. Another man found images of large-breasted women to be tantalizing, and he never went further than his everyday TV shows. Bill found women with long slender necks stimulating. His subway ride back and forth to work was his pornography studio. In the final analysis, pornography is what each man finds stimulating. What stimulates one man may not stimulate another man and vice versa.

While more classifications of pornography exist, pornography is usually found in the following mediums: literature, photos, Internet, sculptures, drawings, paintings, animation, sound recordings, movies, TV, films, DVDs, Blu-ray, pay-for-view, videos, or video games. Let us look at a few of these.

> **Literature and photos:** The spicy novel with sexually stimulating stories and scenes has been around for ages. In the past century, men's magazines such as *Playboy* and *Penthouse* became popular and the source of initiation into the world of sex for many boys. While these magazines do not violate the Supreme Court's standard of obscenity, adult bookstores sell even more sexually explicit magazines that come close to violating the Supreme Court standard of obscenity.

> **Film, DVD, and video:** From the midpoint of the previous century, pornography came off the printed page into movement and even more explicit sexual enactment. Adult bookstores thrived on making available first 8mm movies followed by videocassettes and then DVDs, Blu-rays and intelligent phones. Material sold by adult book stores generally contains hard-core pornography and illicit acts. Adult bookstores look forward to visiting conventioneers who find a trip away from home as an opportunistic time to purchase future pleasure.

TV and pay-for-view: In recent years, the man who subscribes to a full range of cable or satellite TV channels has available more pornography than he could ever digest. The only difficulty he has is finding a time to view his material so he does not get caught. One man said he set his alarm clock for a predawn hour so he could watch sexually stimulating material before going to work. Men who travel frequently may find pay-for-view movies in their hotel room are their downfalls.

Movies: It's difficult to go to a movie theater these days without being exposed to sexually explicit scenes and nudity. While they are acceptable in today's society, they can cause a man to retain images in his head and to mentally process them later, along with masturbation.

Immodest dress: Both women and men dress for attention. Clothing and how it is worn can be alluring or sexually revealing. Young people may or may not recognize that the way they dress will cause sexual arousal—very toxic to a sexually addicted man. One man remarked, "I need blinders when I drive across a college campus. Some young women wear less clothing than allowed in a doctor's exam room."

Internet: The Internet is the ultimate presentation of pornography in today's society. While many web sites entice men to pay for more explicit images, plenty of material is available for free. More disturbing is available material that exploits children. If depression was the mental health common cold of the last century, Internet pornography is the pneumonia of this century. Of greater concern is the number of young people and teenagers who have unfettered access to sexually stimulating material on the Internet.

Cybersex: Cybersex has as its common elements the use of a computer, Internet access, expected anonymity, and sexually provocative material to generate arousal followed most often by masturbation. Multiple venues exist such as dial-a-porn, e-mail, chat rooms, live video streams, instant messaging, postings to social networks, visual images of real or graphically generated persons, and interactive sex through a web cam.

Statistics on pornography

The market for Internet pornography is huge and it is growing. Unfortunately, more children are being exposed to pornography and thus are potential victims of sexual addiction. The following tables give insight into just how insidious just one form of sexual stimulation has become—Internet pornography.

United States Pornography Revenues
Revenue from pornography is more than $97 billion a year. The pornography industry has larger revenues than the revenues of the top technology companies **combined:** Microsoft, Google, Amazon, eBay, Yahoo, Apple, Netflix, and Earthlink. Revenue from pornography in the United States exceeds the combined revenues of ABC, CBS, and NBC

Pornography Time Statistics
Every second—$3,075.64 is spent on pornography
Every second—28,258 Internet users are viewing pornography
Every 39 minutes: a new pornographic video is created in the United States

Internet Pornography Statistics	
Pornographic web sites	4.2 million (12% of total web sites)
Pornographic pages	**420 million**
Daily pornographic search engine requests	68 million (25% of search engine requests)
Daily Gnutella "child pornography" requests	116,000
Web sites offering illegal child pornography	**100,000**
Youths who received sexual solicitation	one in seven

Children Internet Pornography Statistics	
Average age of first Internet exposure to pornography	**11 years-of-age**
15-17 year olds who have multiple hard-core exposures	80%
8-16 year olds who have viewed porn online	**90% (most while doing homework)**

Adult Internet Pornography Statistics	
Percentage of Internet users who view pornography	42.7%
Men admitting to accessing pornography at work	20%
US adults who regularly visit Internet pornography web sites	40 million
Promise Keeper men who viewed pornography in the last week	**53%**
Christians who said pornography is a major problem in the home	**47%**

(Family Safe Media, 2012)

The problem that pornography is causing in our society is staggering and growing. Just think: if while you were at church this past Sunday, you looked left and right, one of the two people you greeted could have said pornography is a problem in their home. If 53% of Promise Keeper men admit to viewing pornography last week, you are far from alone.

Internet pornography content

When one thinks of a man viewing pornography on the Internet, it is reasonable to think of him viewing women in some form of normal sexuality. The reality is the Internet provides both normal sexuality as well as a large menu of perverted sexuality. Briefly, examples of perverted sexual behavior are bestiality, sadomasochism (S & M), sexual violence including sadomasochism and rape, exploitation of children, and other perversions that go beyond the need to describe them here.

A therapist asked the men in his sexual addiction therapy group to disclose the nature of the material they viewed on line. The purpose of asking them to disclose Internet pornography images of choice was to explore a connection between current interests and a disturbing event that occurred during childhood. When such a connection is identified, it may be possible to reduce the addictive power of the current interest.

Glenn's story

Glenn was a city boy who was sent to his uncle's farm one summer when he was about the age of ten. To the farm boy, animal copulation is part of everyday business. His cousin realized that Glenn had never seen animals mate. He took Glenn to the pasture one day when the veterinarian was on hand to breed a stallion with a prized mare. Glenn was not ready for what he witnessed. He was sexually stimulated and confused by seeing the mating process. He remembers dreaming about what he saw a number of times over the next several years. In fact, he became fascinated with human copulation as well.

Glenn, as an adult, stumbled on an Internet site that featured bestiality. He returned to that site and others like it for several years. He never understood why this perverted act stimulated him. While in therapy he was able to see the connection between what happened at age ten and what kept him fixated as an adult.

If you are addicted to Internet pornography, some steps are available to help you. For the man who is not computer savvy, a number of commercial software programs are available to block access to pornography. Type in "blocking software" into your Internet browser search bar and you'll find multiple alternatives.

For the man who is computer savvy enough to get around Internet blocking programs, software entitled *Covenant Eyes* is excellent. This software goes beyond blocking access to web sites the user wishes to access. It provides a weekly report to a person designated by the user to receive the report. The report details every site the user accessed during the week of reference. Covenant Eyes (2012) can be found on http: //www.covenanteyes.com/

Other rather simple changes are also available to you. For example, relocate your computer to a "public area" within your home. Commit not to use your computer when you are "home alone."

Other more stringent solutions to ward off access to pornography include cancelling access to cable TV, not watching any TV show that, in the past, provided stimulating images, cancelling your subscription to certain sports magazines that feature advertizing or articles with tantalizing images, and taping TV shows in order to fast forward past provocative scenes or commercials.

Unfortunately the standard for men who are addicted to pornography is no longer the same as that for the average "Joe." What the average "Joe" can view without sexual interest is far different from that for the man addicted to pornography.

People can't live with change if there's not a changeless core inside them. The key to the ability to change is a changeless sense of who you are, what you are about and what you value.

Stephen Covey

Chapter Five

Codependency

Clinical experience has shown that sexually-addicted men, when they marry, often marry into a codependent relationship. Codependency will affect the marriage and may affect the addict's recovery. Both partners may find it beneficial to examine their role in the marriage.

To begin this chapter, a few thoughts may add clarity:

- The term codependency was first coined in the Alcoholic Anonymous community. As it relates to sexual addiction, I define codependency as the propensity of marriage partners to look for happiness or the lack of contentment based on the behavior of the partner. In simpler terms, each partner expects the other partner to cause their happiness. Melody Beattie (1992), a well known author in the field of codependency defines codependency as:

  A codependent person is one who has let another person's behavior affect him or her, and who is obsessed with controlling that person's behavior.

- For the sexually addicted male, there is a clear road map to codependency. It is almost universal that the sexually addicted man did not have a nourishing relationship with his father—and in some cases, with his mother, when his mother assumed the characteristics of the paternal role in the family. Bradshaw (1988) relates:

  Co-dependence is the most common family illness because it is what happens to anyone in any kind of the dysfunctional family. In every dysfunctional family, there is a primary stressor. This could be Dad's drinking or work addiction; Mom's hysterical control of everyone's feelings; Dad or Mom's physical or verbal violence; a family member's actual sickness or hypochondriasis; Dad or Mom's early death; their divorce; Dad or Mom's moral/religious righteousness; Dad or Mom's sexual abuse. Anyone, who becomes controlling in the family to the point of being experienced as a threat by the other members, initiates the dysfunction.

Again, the vast majority of sexually addicted men grew up in a dysfunctional family, often abusive, and most often with parents who were codependent themselves. It is natural for the sexually addicted man, when he seeks a partner, to find one who also experienced dysfunction and codependency in her family.

Perhaps, as you read Bradshaw's description of codependency you will find elements that relate to you.

Codependency in marriages where the male is sexually addicted

When a sexually addicted man marries into a codependent relationship, his spouse often plays the role of the mother who feels responsible for fixing her child (husband)—a way of controlling him or making herself feel indispensable. Since the man likely did not learn good communication or parenting skills from his family of origin, he gives his spouse plenty of opportunities to tell him about his deficiencies. The addicted man plays the role of the damaged child who needs someone to chastise and fix him. The wife takes the superior position in the marriage and the addicted man takes the subordinate position. The marriage is unbalanced. Mutual respect and acceptance of one another on the basis of equality is absent. Unfortunately, the unbalanced marriage helps to keep the man steeped in his sexual addiction.

Interestingly, the spouse does not see herself in the superior position. She sees herself in the victim position. She sees herself as the recipient of her partner's broken promises to do better, his inability to show affection other than through sex, and his inability to communicate except through anger, etc.

She sees the man whom she thought she loved fail miserably as the husband she thought she married. She keeps trying to help (or fix) him because she craves the husband of her dreams.

Frequently, her family of origin was dysfunctional and did not provide her with the loving nourishment she needed to feel whole. She looked to marriage to fill the gaps in her life. She too is hurting in the marriage. Her need for the husband of her dreams is conditioned by her own insecurity, her own feelings of being abandoned, and her sorrow at not being connected to her husband. Although the above is not a universal characterization of the marriage relationships among all sexually addicted men and their spouses, it is reality for many.

Neither partner is getting what they expected nor what they need from the marriage relationship. His isolation grows and he uses his addiction to medicate his pain of isolation. Her effort to help (or fix) her husband has the exact opposite of her intended effect and she grows more frustrated with his failures.

Who is to blame?

This chapter is not intended to assess blame on one or both partners. It merely conveys the reality that is found in many relationships involving a sexually addicted person. If after you read this chapter, you believe you are in a codependent relationship, then you are fortunate in your recognition. With knowledge comes power, and the choice to change what is not working in your relationship.

To explore how codependency affects marriages where the male is sexually addicted, we have two stories. The stories include many of the characteristics found in codependent relationships.

Codependency characteristics are often evident before marriage

Jim and Barbara's story

Jim dated while he was in high school for social conformity. Since he had not witnessed respectful interactions between his parents, his relationship skills were also lacking. He did not know what it meant to get to know and appreciate a person of the opposite sex. Outside of school dances and similar functions, his social contact focused primarily on "making out." While "making out" never progressed beyond heavy petting, it was not for a lack of desire on his part.

Barbara also dated in high school. The man she dated was several years older and was in the military. For her, the relationship was safe because of the distance and infrequency of face to face contact. Having experienced a dysfunctional family environment, she too lacked understanding of a healthy relationship. She had a sense of loneliness because she often fought with her parents.

Jim and Barbara's parents were alike in many ways. Neither set of parents showed much affection. Jim's father was an alcoholic. Barbara and Jim felt their parents loved them, but external signs of affection were rare. When Jim left for college, the message he believed his parents sent was: anything short of a high level of performance was unacceptable. Barbara's motivation was more based on an internal perception that her parents would not love her if she did not succeed in her academic pursuits.

Barbara and Jim met at a college sponsored mixer for incoming freshman where upperclassmen were invited to attend. Jim felt an immediate attraction to Barbara. To him, she had all the physical attributes that met his criteria for an attractive girl. He felt she was a bit naïve, but thought it was cute. On the other hand, while she thought Jim was reasonably attractive, she was not particularly interested in dating him. She had not planned to get involved with a college man because her studies were more important to her.

Jim invited Barbara to campus social affairs and fraternity parties. The first several times she turned him down. She finally agreed to go to a fraternity mixer. By this time, Jim was sexually attracted to Barbara. In fact, he had a number of erotic dreams that included Barbara. Jim began to plot ways to manipulate Barbara into a sexual relationship to satisfy his needs. Several months after their initial encounter, their relationship turned sexual. Once sexual activity entered into their relationship, neither seemed to put a priority on developing a strong non-sexual friendship. The glue that held the relationship together was physical and emotional dependency on each other.

Jim and Barbara dated for several years before they married. During this time, Jim's sexual needs continued to grow while Barbara tried to satisfy her need to be loved by giving into Jim's need.

Codependency characteristics flourish in marriage

Jim and Barbara married and began a family. A year or so into the marriage, it became very apparent to Barbara that Jim was very self-centered and manipulative. His needs always seemed to come first. Joint decisions were often the product of Jim's persuasion. While he was a good economic provider, as a loving companion, he was far from ideal. Barbara felt very alone in the marriage and focused all her attention on raising their children. She tried numerous times to talk to him about her needs and her perception of a loving marriage. He repeatedly made promises to do better but did not do so. His perception was, as long as he provided a good economic subsistence for the family, he fulfilled his end of the bargain. Because he felt that Barbara constantly suggested ways in which he needed to improve, he shied away from give and take discussions because he feared he would see himself as a failure. Jim and Barbara grew apart in their marriage.

More than a decade into their marriage, Barbara learned that Jim had been unfaithful. Jim had marital affairs with several women at work and was addicted to pornography. In one long evening he confessed all of his transgressions and begged for Barbara's forgiveness. Jim insisted he would become a new man. Jim initially felt relieved that his greatest and most shameful secrets were exposed. The stress of leading a secret, dual life had become almost intolerable.

His promise to become a new man was short lived. He kept a secret stash of pornographic material for his periodic fix. In the deep recesses of his mind he reasoned he could, as he had done in the past, manipulate Barbara into accepting his promise to change his ways—and move on. Not this time! Barbara now recognized his manipulative behavior, and was not satisfied with his explanations, or his promises. Barbara was angry and decided she was not going to let Jim get away with what he had done to her and their family.

She embarked on a plan to hold him accountable to his promise to change his behavior.

Jim wondered if the cure was not worse than the disease. He contemplated leaving Barbara but was terrified with the thought of being alone and isolated from his children. He hoped that Barbara's fury would abate with time, but he was wrong.

Barbara also wondered whether she wanted to stay in the marriage. "Was it worth it," she asked herself? She contemplated leaving Jim, but was confounded by the thought of being financially insecure, and having to raise the children by herself. She convinced herself to stay until the children were in college. She made plans to get a job so she could grow financially independent. She saw Jim as a selfish "bastard" who was out to get his sexual needs met notwithstanding the total disregard for the marriage covenant. While she did not put it in terms of "punishment," she felt he had it coming when she monitored his every move. She had given up hope of ever trusting him again. And yet, deep down she felt she needed him and the security that he provided. She saw Jim as a pathetic sex monger and herself as the victim of his total selfishness.

Jim and Barbara's marriage had hit rock bottom. Both were very angry people living under the same roof and incapable of seeing a way out of their dysfunctional relationship.

Epilog

Jim and Barbara were living in a codependent destructive world. Both were living under false premises. Jim thought his future happiness lay in Barbara agreeing to love him for whom he was without her trying to change him. Barbara saw her future happiness as a product of a reinvented Jim, and she was going to take charge of his reinventing.

Barbara was not going to be successful in changing Jim. Only Jim could change Jim. Sex could no longer be his greatest need. Jim's good friend suggested he consider getting help. On his own volition, Jim entered sex addiction counseling and participated in an accompanying Twelve Step program. Jim's healing would take time and he would have to grieve the damage he had done to himself, and to all those around him.

Marital therapy would be needed to reestablish trust, friendship, and a spiritual connection in the marriage. The healing journey will take years. Since Jim and Barbara contemplated divorce, if they don't invest fully in the therapy program, they are doomed to repeat the same failures in any subsequent marriage. Ultimately, with therapy and commitment they can find the relationship both want and need in their present marriage.

Codependency characteristics in Jim and Barbara's marriage

The following are characteristics of codependency found in Jim and Barbara's story. You may or may not find yourselves in their story, but the principles set below mirrors the experiences of many couples where the male is sexually addicted.

Characteristic # 1

The origin of codependency is found in a child's dysfunctional family

Parents of codependent children are often codependent themselves, as were Jim and Barbara's parents. The traits are handed down, that is, taught to each succeeding generation. The parents of the codependent children are ill equipped to provide emotional nourishment to their children. Instead, dysfunctional families abound in addiction, narcissism, and the inability to show love to their children. When parents are internally focused on their own problems, they are ill equipped to build healthy relationships with their children. They can't give what they don't have.

Jim's father was an alcoholic. As such, he was not aware of the developmental needs of his son. Jim learned from his father how to be self-centered. He learned that earning his father's love was based on his performance. His father looked to Jim to succeed where he himself had failed. Jim's mother was a codependent enabler of her husband's alcoholism; that is, she continued to purchase alcohol for her husband. Jim could not get his emotional needs met from his family of origin. While he was unable to codify it as a child, as an adult he recognized that he was emotionally abandoned by his parents. His emotional deficiency led him to focus on satisfying his needs without regard to the needs of those around him.

From his parents, Jim also learned to manipulate others into meeting his needs. He used dominance to trump normal healthy interactions in his relationships. He was unable to be a friend and have empathy for others.

Jim was also sexually abused as a child at the hands of an older sibling. As he grew older, he turned to sexual stimulation for feelings of well being. He substituted sexual satisfaction for friendship and respect in his relationships.

Barbara's father was emotionally distant from his family. His work and weekend golf took precedence over his family. If he had a choice, he chose to be absent from his wife and children. When Barbara was a teenager, her mother often talked about wanting to leave her husband, but never did so. Barbara now recognizes that her parents were in a codependent relationship. Barbara did not experience a sense of well being from her parents. She felt she had to earn parental love. Among her siblings, she was the caretaker and the responsible child.

Both Jim and Barbara were predestined to enter into a codependent relationship.

Characteristic # 2

Children of codependent dysfunctional families have ill-formed or incomplete personalities

Adult behavior, either intentionally or not, builds on the dysfunctional personality traits learned in the family of origin.

Jim often felt deficient in his social skills, and questioned his self-worth. Because of his low self-esteem, he often wondered if anyone really could love him. Nevertheless, his distorted thinking led him to equate sex with a feeling of being loved. Through his previous experience with sexual stimulation, he sought mood escalation by repeated attempts to manipulate his high school and college girl friends. It never occurred to Jim that there was much more to a relationship than making out. After all, he reasoned, if a girl would participate in sexual activity with him, surely they loved each other.

Barbara's hole in the soul was her need to be loved. In response to the attention she received from Jim, she allowed herself to be manipulated into an early sexual relationship. From time to time, she felt sex occupied far too much of their relationship. Several times she attempted to establish what she considered more healthy boundaries. She was no match for Jim's manipulative skills.

Jim's attraction to Barbara focused on her attractive body parts. He lacked the insight needed to focus on her personality and her personhood. He felt that the essence of a steady relationship was to have Barbara depend on him. While Barbara frequently felt uneasy, she also lacked the skills to objectively evaluate their relationship. She bought into depending on him for an active college environment. After all, he was a fraternity brother and she wore his pin.

Characteristic # 3

In marriage, codependency fosters pain and negativity

Once married, Jim's eyes began to wander. He needed the thrill of pursuing a new conquest. He began to repeat the cycle he began with Barbara while they were in college. Jim lacked marriage skills and his pursuits outside of the marriage bed further distanced him from providing the emotional nourishment Barbara so dearly needed.

Barbara substituted her desire for marital happiness by focusing her attention on her children. Her friends saw her as an outstanding and dedicated mother. She tried to meet her children's every need. Barbara transferred her dependence on Jim to dependence on her children for her emotional well being. She tried to fill the hole in her soul by forming a loving relationship with her children. However, children are unable to return love as would a healthy adult.

Jim continued to insist on sex with Barbara, who was fearful of saying no because she feared Jim's anger. Barbara felt disconnected from Jim. She gave him what he wanted but she felt she was simply paying dues.

Characteristic # 4

Fear, shame, anger, and depressed mood are all companions of codependency

Jim continued to live in two worlds—one foot in his sexual fantasy world and one foot inside the home. While he believed he was clever enough to not get caught, he realized that his life was out of control, and getting worse. He was ashamed and lived in a low-grade depressed mood. He knew that his relationship with Barbara had gone from good to bad but had no idea how to change it. He had no intention of giving up his best friend, sex. After all, as many sexually addictive men reason, a man needs some pleasure in life.

When Barbara learned of Jim's closely-held secrets, she felt conflicting emotions. On the one hand, she was relieved that her suspicions were real and she was not crazy. On the other hand, she was outraged, and felt great anger. She was also dominated by fear. She was fearful she would be left totally alone in life: what would become of her and the children? How could anyone understand the intense feeling of betrayal she felt? She was so depressed that getting out of bed each day, eating, and caring for the children seemed like monumental tasks.

Characteristic # 5

Codependency is part of the problem

For Jim and Barbara, codependency was an integral part of their marriage. Jim depended on his ability to manipulate Barbara so he could continue to get his needs met. Barbara depended on her anger to respond to Jim's betrayal of their marriage contract.

Neither would be successful.

Both would benefit from counseling. Jim needed to address his addictive behavior. Barbara would have done well to seek counseling to heal the consequences of her marital relationship. They both needed help to deal with the present crisis, and to help support the family.

Joe and Alice's story

Joe, a mid-level executive, had multiple affairs during his twenty years of marriage to Alice. It was usual for Joe to have more than one affair going at the same time. While his marriage to Alice provided him with two wonderful children, he continued his liaisons. He said, "I don't feel particularly close to Alice. She does her thing, and I do mine."

Joe protected his computer and e-mail account with passwords. One evening he inadvertently left his e-mail account open. Alice stumbled onto Joe's e-mail exchanges with his ladies. Pandemonium ensued.

Alice went to Joe and demanded full disclosure. Joe complied but refused to give sufficient details to satisfy Alice. Joe felt he did not want to cause more pain than he had already caused. He also talked about the shame of his behavior and his fear that Alice would leave him if she knew the details. Alice wanted a full accounting of all his transgressions and she wanted him to keep her abreast of his behavior and thinking on a daily basis. She was angry and terrified. She felt betrayed, and was concerned about the future of their marriage and the raising of their children.

Neither Joe nor Alice wanted a divorce but the bond between them had been fractured. Joe said that for years he wanted to let Alice in on his most guarded secrets of infidelity, but feared she would try to fix him or leave him. In fact, his fears became a reality. Alice, in her despondency, did everything she could think of to hold Joe accountable to her perception of a good marriage. In her zeal to monitor Joe, she obtained his credit card and telephone records for as many years as she could. On a continuing basis, she questioned any call that was not readily recognizable. She constantly accused him of going back to being unfaithful. She insisted on obtaining the phone number for each of the women with whom he had been unfaithful. She called every one of them to make it clear that Joe was no longer available. She embarrassed him by talking about what a rotten person he was to anyone who would listen—at his work, church, and community.

Alice continued to demand more information and frequently asked questions about one or more of his affairs. Periodically Joe would provide the detail of an affair which then resulted in Alice's berating him for the content of the detail. After each disclosure, she yelled that she could not trust him, because she did not know how much more he had not told her.

They discussed their behavior in a joint marital therapy session. Alice and Joe made promises to change, but they did not. Their marriage therapist speculated that Alice had a hole in her soul related to sexual abuse as a child. In other words, she had her own shame. Shame binds Joe to Alice. Unless they deal with the roots of their dysfunction from childhood, it is unlikely the marriage will survive.

The other side of the coin

Perhaps you have experienced the same steps that Alice took to reclaim her partner. Do you agree that there was nothing wrong with her taking positive action? Why shouldn't she demand accountability? Why shouldn't she demand that you confess your transgressions in real time so she could know how sincere you were in your promise to change? After all, she is the victim of your profound selfishness—putting your needs ahead of everything dear and sacred to the marriage contract.

The answer?

Alice is justified in her anger. However, if Joe is not committed to hold himself accountable to changing his behavior, Alice's efforts are headed for frustration and divorce. It is Joe who has to see that putting his sexual needs ahead of all else has a dim future.

Alice's actions add to Joe's shame. Sexual addiction is a shame-based disease. While hardly an excuse to justify acting-out behavior, shame and feelings of worthlessness often contribute to acting out. Sexually addicted men self medicate negative feelings. One of the tasks sexually addicted men address during recovery is exposing their sense of shame to the light of day. Group and Twelve Step programs seek to counter negativity which exist in their lives. An essential step is to learn to take positive steps to come out of isolation, allowing shame to recede, and to forgo living in low-grade depression. Perhaps one could argue that Joe deserves to feel guilt and shame but doing so will not help him on his recovery journey.

A visual picture of Joe and Alice's codependency relationship

Picture two elevators side by side: Joe occupies one and Alice the other. When Alice's elevator is on the tenth floor, Joe's elevator is in the basement. When Joe's elevator is in the basement, he sees himself as the errant child and he looks up to Alice on the tenth floor and sees a scornful mother. Joe gives Alice the power to chastise, for he believes he deserves it, but he intensely resents her for doing so. Alice takes the power given to her and dutifully scolds and punishes. She is no longer the spouse, but has taken the role of Jim's dysfunctional mother.

They ride their elevators to the opposite levels. Alice's elevator is now in the basement and Joe's is on the tenth floor. Alice sees herself as the victim of Joe's self-centeredness. She sees his behavior as willful, destructive to the marriage, and selfish. She sees him in a superior position—doing his own thing without regard to the consequences, particularly to the marriage. Joe supports her vision by continuing to put his sexual needs first.

Joe and Alice continue to ride their respective elevators, alternating between the basement and tenth floor. As they ride, they get more and more angry, and blame each other for their predicament.

What needs to change?

In simplistic terms, both Joe and Alice would do well to ride their elevators to the fifth floor, get off, and face one another.

Ideally, Joe admits he is powerless to stop his behavior—it has become unmanageable.

Alice rejects the role of Joe's mother. Alice tells Joe, "It is not my job to change you. That is your challenge." If so inclined, she can tell him, "I will pray for you. If you would like a friendly ear while you are in therapy, I may agree to listen, but I am not willing to try to be your accountability partner or make suggestions."

Alice may choose to deal with the origins of her codependent behavior in individual or group therapy.

Joe's fifth floor position is to thank Alice and to commit to counseling. His therapist will likely also recommend he attend one or multiple Twelve Step programs on a regular basis.

You and codependency addressed

In a healthy marriage, partners see themselves neither in a superior position nor as the victim, but as equals. Each takes individual responsibility to grow in wisdom. Your goal, as the addict, is to accept that you have a problem which you commit to address. The wife's goal is to accept that she, too, has issues that she could address. The two of you support each other in a quest to become whole, and shun the paralyzing effects of shame.

In a codependent relationship, each partner's identity lies outside of the self. Each depends on the other to provide wholeness. Neither partner is independent in the relationship. For example, if you would like to change your partner's behavior, you are saying, "For me, happiness lies in how my partner can change, not on how I function independently." In a codependent relationship, both parties want to be in charge but neither party feels that they are, and yet, each party feels the other is in charge.

A practical way to change your codependent response is: instead of giving advice, ask your partner how she is dealing with such and such a situation. Thank her for her thoughts. Assure her you are committed to work on your issues. Tell her you are open to hear what she has learned and interested in what she wants to share. Don't let yourself engage in a codependent response.

If your partner attempts to give you advice, ask her to tell you how it would change her if you followed her advice. Thank her for sharing, and tell her that you need to ponder what you heard. You are now free to either make the change or not. Just because someone wants something, that doesn't mean they are going to get it. However, respond in love! Don't be dead right! The difference in the above behavior is: you have introduced loving independence.

Note: Your partner did not cause your addiction nor did codependency. Your addiction began long before you met your partner and before codependency entered your lives. Banish the thought of blaming your partner's codependency on your addiction. The reason for providing a detailed description of codependency is to help you understand that a loving and joyful marriage in the future will depend on ridding your marriage of <u>both</u> addiction and codependency.

Anger will never disappear so long as thoughts of resentment are cherished in the mind. Anger will disappear just as soon as thoughts of resentment are forgotten.

Buddha

Chapter Six

Role of Anger, Anxiety, and Depression

Perhaps you have concluded that unwanted sexual behavior is part of your life. Do you also feel angry but do not know why? Do you often find yourself feeling somewhat depressed or anxious? You are not alone! These three emotional states, anxiety, anger, and depressed mood, often accompany and contribute to unwanted sexual behaviors and sexual addiction. All three of these emotional states are companions of men who sexually act out.

Role of Anger

Childhood abuse

Often the roots of anger are formed in childhood. When a child does not receive the emotional nourishment he needs, he often thinks that the problem is within him. It is rare for a young boy to understand that the problem is with his parents. If a young child could believe his parents are defective, this dependant child would experience an overwhelming feeling of isolation. Thus, the child often thinks he is defective or bad.

John Bradshaw's (1988) words bear repeating:

> . . . [If] parents are abusive and hurt the child through physical, sexual, emotional or mental pain, the child will assume the blame, make himself bad, in order to keep all-powerful protection against the terrors of night. For a child at this stage to realize the inadequacies of parents would produce unbearable anxiety.

What does a child do when he thinks he is to blame and considers himself bad? For many, the child develops two images or faces of himself. The face he presents to the world is the person he wants the world to view. This is the good self. This is the self who achieves, who appears happy, who obeys the rules. The other face is that of the bad or defective child. When sexual abuse is present, the bad self is convinced of his intrinsic evil and feels profound shame. He is very fearful that others might see his bad face and goes to great lengths to hide it. He isolates his bad self, builds a wall around it, and never talks to his parents or another adult about being sexual. He internalizes his shameful feelings.

The child believes he has a need to project a good face while feeling intrinsically that the good face is not the real self. The child defends the good self and fears exposure of the defective self. This model of good and defective selves grows with the child and eventually becomes part of the adult life.

When the adult thinks that another person or experience may expose the defective self, the natural reaction is fear. Fear is externalized as anger, anxiety, or depression.

For example, it is relatively common for a child to believe that parents expect perfect behavior. The child learns to value performance and thinks the way to earn love is to be perfect. As an adult, being perfect recalls childhood messages. Although the adult wants the world to believe that he is perfect, the wounded self knows that being perfect is just a front—inside the adult knows he is far from perfect. When another person pierces the mask of perfect and touches the fearful inner soul, anger results.

Ralph's story

Ralph explained, "My thinking is not always logical. When someone cuts me off in traffic, I internalize it as though they were saying, 'You are less important, less worthy of the space on the road.' I just fume when I feel I am devalued. When I hit a bad golf shot, my feelings of being a flawed person are exposed. If I were the good golfer—the good person—I would not hit bad shots. I get so angry when I hit bad shots that I teach the world around me new words."

Ralph's anger is not in proportion to the importance of the events. It is triggered by his perception of being devalued or flawed. As he increases awareness of his anger triggers, Ralph begins to understand that he has the choice of changing his thinking. He talks about his two faces. He thinks that his anger would be less if his two faces became congruent, came together. He says the first step in healing his two faces is to acknowledge that in reality the bad self is a fraud. In fact, like other sincere people, he is on a journey. Ralph begins to understand, "Bad is part of life . . . it is not who I am."

With this insight he reported on his next golf game. "I was less angry this past Monday when I hit bad shots. I did not verbalize my anger as much but I was still angry. It will take time to become aware 'in the present moment' of my underlying feelings of inadequacy before I react in anger. My new experience would go something like this. Hit bad shot, feel distress, anger. Before reacting

I say to myself, 'You hit a bad shot. Lots of folks hit bad shots. Hitting a bad shot does not mean I am a bad person. Relax. Now hit a good shot.'"

Men who feel bad and defective because they sexually act out need to reevaluate their thinking. Let them understand that although they judge acting out behavior to be bad, it does not mean they are bad people. There is an important difference between bad behavior and being intrinsically bad or evil. God does not create evil people. He does create people who can make bad choices. Peter was told to forgive seventy times seven. God's standard is to forgive every time we ask to be forgiven. If God does not condemn the sinner, is it not folly for men to condemn themselves? So, replace your "bad self" thinking with the Twelve Step thought: "I am powerless over my bad behavior, but I will take the steps to get help and learn to choose to change."

Childhood messages

Although the concept of two faces, good and bad self surely does not fit all who feel angry, those with anger concerns are well served to think back to childhood to find their anger roots. What messages did you receive as a child from parents, siblings, and childhood friends? How did you feel about those messages? Are you still fearful of those messages? Are the negative feelings ingrained during your childhood the underlying source of your adult anger?

Some common messages sent by dysfunctional parents are:

- It is not safe to express your feelings.

- We will love you only if you do well in school or sports.

- There is no time for play around here. You need to fix dinner and take care of your siblings.

- You are a failure!

- Your opinion doesn't count in this house. I will tell you what to think!

- You need to be the man of the house.

- Bs on your report card are not good enough. You can do better.

- You will never measure up to our expectations.

- I will give you something to cry about.

- You are bad just like your father.

- You couldn't possibly amount to anything.

- Children are to be seen, not heard.

- Why can't you be like your older siblings?

Each of these statements is harsh and negative. Each expresses a judgment. The child learns that love is conditional. He is not a person of worth. Life is negative. Negative feelings lead to negative judgments about self. If a child does not feel the joy of being loved unconditionally, chances are he will respond to life on the opposite side of the spectrum—in anger.

Rules in the head

Messages, like those above, form the basis for a person's rules of life. If the rules taught to the child are negative, the rules an adult forms for his own behavior and for the behavior of others similarly will be negative. Chances are that he will form a rather comprehensive set of negative and harsh rules that he expects himself and all others to obey. Because he tends to be isolated, he will not share the rules in his head with those around him. However, his rules for their behavior are his standards and he expects himself and others to follow them.

Sean's story

Sean carried many rules around in his head. He said, "I believe that we must have order. For example, I have a real thing about shopping carts left around parking lots. All shopping carts must be returned to their proper place. One day I drove into the grocery parking lot and observed another patron, who had emptied his cart, abandon it in the parking space to which I was heading. I stopped my truck right in the middle of the parking lot, got out, and proceeded to lambaste the poor fellow. In retrospect, I think my anger was out of proportion. But he had it coming, didn't he? I wonder why this rule in my head is so important to me?"

Sean harbors many other rules in his head. Others don't know Sean's rules. He keeps them locked in his brain. Yet Sean expects others to know the rules of his game. Others constantly violate Sean's rules. It is not difficult to see that Sean is an angry man—people constantly violate the rules in his head. How could they not?

Anger at God

Many men who are addicted, express anger at God. Their thinking may be:

- Why did He let this happen to me?

- A loving God would not permit evil, death, and suffering.

- I have prayed for years for God to take away my unwanted sexual behavior but He hasn't listened to me. The Bible says my prayers are heard. Maybe so, but I think my prayers have not been answered.

- If God really loved me, He would take away my illness.

- Why do bad things always happen to me? Where is God when I need Him?

Being angry with God, paradoxically, is an expression of love for God. When we are angry at God, our anger is an affirmation of God's importance in our lives. It is all right to be angry with God. However, it is prudent to examine our anger logic. Anger at God is often a result of faulty expectations of what we can rightfully expect from Him, given that His most precious gift to us is free will. Is God's answer to you, "I loved you so much I have given you the power to make choices?" Spiritual counseling often helps us to think more clearly.

Anger alters mood

The underlying principle of sexual addiction is mood alteration. When a man engages in his acting out ritual and subsequently acts out, his mood is temporarily lifted. He escapes his pain. Interestingly, anger can also be used to alter mood. Men report feeling a rush during a fit of rage. Thus, the buildup and the outburst of anger have similar characteristics to the sexual ritual and subsequent acting out. Arnie reported that when he became sexually sober he believed that his outbursts of anger increased. This did not make sense to him. He thought sexual sobriety would bring him peace. When he got in touch with how he felt when he experienced rage, he began to see that he substituted one form of mood altering for another.

Role of Anxiety

Anxiety is a state of emotional discomfort, one in which a person often feels a sense of inability to manage a situation or event. An anxious person may be fearful that something is going to happen—often bad. There is a pervasive feeling of uneasiness or apprehension.

Although the clinical definition does not address the relationship between anxiety and unwanted sexual behavior, stories from those in sexual addiction therapy reveal a strong connection. The link between anxiety and unwanted sexual behavior is so strong that dealing with anxiety is a very important step on the road to recovery.

Sexual anxiety

For some men visual stimulation creates significant sexual tension. Once a man sees an attractive person or sexual material, a physical response is triggered in his body. It is different from just being aroused. Men, who experience sexual anxiety, often have great difficulty concentrating, feel restless, and cannot perform normal daily functions. The anxiety affects work performance, family, or other life responsibilities. However, the symptom most compelling is a strong feeling of muscle tension in the genital area that does not initially include an erection. The tension is disturbing. It stays with him despite his efforts to change thinking or activity.

Barry's story

Barry is a student. He said, "During the warm months, the young women on campus dress, you know, very casually. Even in class I am often distracted by the amount of uncovered flesh. It is really hard for me to concentrate. God knows I want to forgo my sexual behavior, but I often come back to my room from class in a state of sexual tension. My whole body aches. I feel as if my genital area is on fire. I feel tense and ready to respond. I hate to fight the battle—to act out or not to give in. It just seems that often I am unsuccessful in moving onto other activities until I relieve these feelings."

The locus of Barry's anxiety is his genitals. He cannot concentrate on other normal activities until he relieves the sexual anxiety he feels in his genital area.

Situational anxiety

Sexually addicted men often react to their environment. A particular situation will trigger a feeling of a desire to act out. Whenever the situation is repeated, they exhibit anxiety symptoms and are unable to function normally. They become tense, irritable, unable to think clearly, and obsessed with relieving their situational anxiety.

Todd's Story

Todd talks about growing up, saying, "My father was a doctor and my mother taught chemistry at the university. I was always exposed to books and our dinner table conversation was like a seminar—very high level conversation. By the time I was five, I had read several of Dad's Hardy Boys books. My parents picked my preschool, kindergarten, and elementary schools so that I could attend the best high school in town. They said my going to the best schools would improve my chances to go to Harvard or Yale. From the earliest days, I knew that anything other than a top performance in school was unacceptable."

Todd inherited his parents' intellect, but he fell into the habit of procrastination. He says, "While in grade school and high school, procrastination never hurt me. I got excellent grades. I went on to a top Ivy League school. I found I was now competing with the cream of the crop—others who were as bright as me. Unfortunately, I brought along my propensity to procrastinate. The consequence was a fear that I might not get all my work done and fail to get top honors."

"The anxiety I felt as I finally sat down to study each night, usually around midnight, was intense. I found I could dispel my anxiety by relieving myself. After I masturbated, I could concentrate. If I did not act out, I was miserable. I never felt the desire to masturbate unless my anxiety was at its peak."

Todd habitually reacted to the situation created by procrastination. He had taught his body to need a physical release. As long as Todd continued to procrastinate, his unwanted sexual behavior would continue. To end his unwanted sexual behavior, Todd first had to understand why he procrastinates. After a period of counseling, Todd decided to address new behaviors to change his procrastination response.

Chronic anxiety

For some men anxiety becomes a way of life. Their lives are dominated by anxiety. They live in a constant state of unrest and a pervasive feeling of uneasiness or apprehension. Surviving each day is a formidable task.

Mack's story

Mack thought that his nickname was a curse. He said, "I never felt like macho Mack. My dad began to call me Mack when I was young. He would say, 'Where is my Mack truck?' I was not a Mack truck. I was Matthew! I grew up feeling like life was going to hand me a bad deal. I constantly felt uneasy and apprehensive. I was sure that, given the opportunity to succeed, I could pluck defeat out of the jaws of victory. Dad thought so too. He constantly told me how much I disappointed him."

Mack was sexually abused by Benjamin, a family member. The abuse continued throughout his childhood years.

Mack, also said, "I lived in fear of Benjamin who told me I had the body and face of a pretty girl. And they called me Mack? I felt sad and angry. Why did I have fine features? Was it my fault that Benjamin always found me when no one else was around? I was afraid to tell Mom or Dad about him. I was sure Dad would tan my hide so I could never sit again. To top it all, I began to stutter. Stuttering just seemed to make matters worse for me. School kids taunted me, 'Pretty boy—talk like a girl.' I felt ashamed and no good."

Life got even worse for Mack. Around age ten he began to wet the bed at night. "Dad really yelled at me when he found out I wet the bed one night. He called me a sissy. I had to hide my problem from him. I found a big piece of plastic to put on my bed on top of the sheets. I was able to awaken as I felt wet and the problem ended."

But Mack's problems continued.

"In high school I was a loner and would masturbate frequently, just like Benjamin had taught me. I dropped out of college after my first year. I found a job in a video store. I lost that job because I could not concentrate and was irritable. I came to work late because I had difficulty sleeping. Masturbation was the only fun I had."

Mack was diagnosed with a generalized anxiety disorder and is in therapy.

Mack's unfortunate life experiences taught him not to trust himself or anyone else. He was totally isolated in his pain and anxiety. He would first have to address his childhood experiences. He would have to internalize that others had hurt him. He had no choice in the events that had shaped him. He would need the guidance of a skilled therapist to help him rethink his life perspective and to begin to understand that he is a person of worth who could make new choices as an adult. Both his anxiety and masturbation are chronic. Only after Mack is able to see outside the wall he has built to protect himself from pain will he begin to defuse his chronic anxiety.

Carnes (2010) frames the issue of the effect of sexual abuse:

> Abuse and neglect deepen this distrust of others and further distort reality. Children who are neglected conclude they are not valuable. In addition, they live with a high level of anxiety because no one teaches them common life skills or provides for their basic needs. Children find ways to deaden the anxiety they inevitably feel, and they do so compulsively. For sex addicts, compulsive masturbation is a good example of an anxiety-reduction strategy. Food and alcohol can be controlled by parents, but it is difficult to stop a young person from masturbating. Other forms of physical and sexual abuse intensify poor self-esteem and the need for relief from fear.

Treatment

Barry, Todd, and Mack all suffer from anxiety, which is related to their sexual behavior. Both their anxieties as well as their unwanted sexual behavior need to be addressed in therapy. When anxiety is the primary condition and sexually acting out is the medication of choice, the underlying cause of anxiety needs to be addressed first. For most, unless the roots of their anxiety are laid bare and pruned, little progress with unwanted sexual behavior will be made. Anti-anxiety medication may also help.

Role of Depressed Mood

Everyone experiences disappointment, failure, and the feeling of abandonment. A student may be disappointed in himself for failing to study sufficiently to get a good grade on an exam. A man may feel a sense of abandonment when his wife chooses to spend the weekend with her friend rather than with him (notwithstanding the compassionate reason his wife has to help her friend). It is a normal function of life to have a bad day. The man with a perpetual smile on his face and an upbeat comment is either a saint or hiding behind a mask. For most, with time and perhaps a little comfort from a friend or family member, the depressed mood passes. Healthy men who experience normal bad days do not use sexual behavior to change their mood.

Chronic depressed mood

Speaking broadly, unwanted sexual behavior usually begins in childhood. For most, the combination of a dysfunctional family environment and exposure to age-inappropriate sexual material or behavior is the root of sexual addiction.

A key element in depression is the dysfunctional family in which the needs of the child for love and affirmation were not met. Not only can this environment lead to inappropriate sexual behavior, it often leads to living in a chronic state of depressed mood. Sexual behavior is a form of self-medication used to raise mood.

The mental health community calls chronically depressed mood a Dysthymic Disorder. Dysthymia is characterized as a depressed mood lasting at least two years during which the person experiences a continuous feeling of malaise (American Psychiatric Association, 2000). Not much in life is going great but, at the same time, one is not so deeply depressed that he cannot function. Perhaps another appropriate descriptive term is low-grade depression.

Those who experience low-grade depression often have low energy, low self-esteem, and a general feeling of hopelessness. Sexual addicts who are also depressed do not feel good about themselves. They are aware that they live behind a mask of respectability but feel deep inside they are terribly flawed.

Perhaps a visual tool will help to explain how low grade depression relates to acting out. This visual tool is called The Addict's Life Scale. This scale ranges from zero to fifty, in ten-point increments. Each benchmark on the scale correlates with a relative mood level. Let's start at the top of the scale and work our way down. The first benchmark on the scale, shown on the following pages, is the fifty-point benchmark. This level signifies the mood associated with acting-out behavior and the feeling of euphoria one feels during the build-up and orgasm. By frequently repeating his acting-out ritual, the addicted man may try to maintain life at the fifty-point benchmark. Let's call this level the "euphoric level."

However, sustaining life at the fifty-point benchmark is difficult because of the shame and guilt that follow acting-out behavior. It becomes a futile chase for the impossible.

One step down, we signify the forty-point benchmark as the normal functioning level. It is the mood level of solid strength and energy. Let's call this level the "Great to be alive" mood level. A recovering addict can see that the margin of difference between the forty-point benchmark and the fifty-point benchmark, his former acting-out behavior level, is only one step, or ten-points away. A man who chooses to live at the "Great to be alive" (forty-point) benchmark, begins to understand that a ten-point gain by acting out is not worth the shame, anger, and discomfort associated with the fifty-point benchmark.

The next step down is the thirty-point benchmark. It is a level below the "Great to be alive" mood level. Let's call this level the "Bad day level." A person who regularly functions at the forty-point benchmark realizes that life has its ups and downs, and it is okay to be down for a short period of time. A person who normally lives at the forty-point benchmark realizes that the thirty-point benchmark is a level he visits, but he does not live there.

The twenty-point benchmark constitutes a low-grade depressed mood or a Dysthymic Disorder level. For most sexually addicted men it is the mood level that accompanies awakening each morning. Life is simply not meeting expectations. One man said, "I got in a rut and I furnished it!" When asked, the sexually addicted man talks about unfulfilled relationships with parents, siblings, and, in particular, his spouse. He has few, if any, close friends. He feels lonely much of the time. He looks for more from life but does not seem to ever find it. He finds he procrastinates because he fears failure.

Profound feelings of shame haunt him. The tone with which he describes himself has elements of "poor me." Other men suffering this low-grade level of depression use the cliché, "Life is a bitch and then you die."

The twenty-point benchmark is a dangerous level. The sexually addicted man sees acting out as an easy way to increase his mood (a thirty-point jump). He will rationalize his acting-out behavior just to "feel better." Men who live at the twenty-point benchmark live in constant low-grade pain. Their underlying discomfort with life is always nagging at their brains. Society teaches us that when we are in pain, we are entitled to take medicine to relieve the pain, and for the addict that medication is acting out sexually.

In this way, the recovering addict who maintains life at a 20-point benchmark is far more susceptible to slipping back into acting-out behavior.

The ten-point benchmark represents full-scale depressed mood. This person finds it difficult to eat, sleep, and to go about daily life. Sexually addicted men rarely experience full-scale depressed mood. They are survivors, and although they do not feel good about themselves, they tend to weather life's daily blows. However, public discovery, particularly when there are legal or divorce implications, is an exception to the survivor mode for the sexually addicted man, and full-scale depression may follow. When the mask comes off, when the deficient self is exposed, friends and relatives often express critical judgments. Those who he once thought would support him often shun the addict most. For the addict's family and acquaintances, the sudden contrast between the person publicly portrayed and the addict's real self is a shocking contradiction that takes time and understanding to resolve.

The zero-point benchmark represents institutionalization. The man who finds himself at the zero-point benchmark is no longer in control of his life. He is not capable of making rational decisions. Other than to identify this level on the scale, it will not be addressed further.

With this introduction, let's look at the Addict's Life Scale.

Addict's Life Scale

50—Acting-out mood. The feeling of euphoria one feels during the build-up and experience of an orgasm.

40—Normal Functioning Mood. The ideal mood level of a normally functioning adult. It is the "great to be alive" mood level.

30—Bad Day Mood. A level to visit but not to stay or live.

20—Low-grade Depressed Mood or Dysthymic Disorder. Where most addicts live life.

10—Full Scale Depressed Mood. The person barely functions.

0—Unable to Function Mood. The person is often institutionalized.

The most important element of the Addict's Life Scale is the thirty-point contrast between the twenty-point benchmark, low-grade depressed mood, and the fifty-point benchmark, the acting-out mood. When the addict chooses the fifty-point benchmark, a thirty-point gain, he feels a sense of euphoria, a high, a rush. The orgasm is the end product. It is the goal; it is the relief from life's pain. His pain is so unacceptable he is willing to go for the short-term fix.

He tells himself:

- I need this!

- I can't live without my fix.

- Life is a bear. I deserve this to be happy once in awhile.

- I earned it!

- Oh, the hell with it, I am going for it!

The key for the addict is to begin to change his life so that the forty-point benchmark the "great to be alive" mood level, becomes more of the norm than the twenty-point benchmark, low-grade depressed mood. Men who make the effort to change how they live so as to experience frequent forty-point level, "great to be alive," feelings, find that a ten-point differential is not enough of a reward to offset the negative consequences of acting out.

Your Addict's Life Scale

How does the Addict's Life Scale apply to your life? At what mood level do you awaken each day? Do you know why you live at that level? What activities or changes can you make to experience the forty-point benchmark level more often? Take a few minutes to record your experience on the Addict's Life Scale below.

50—Acting-out mood.

_____

_____

_____

40—Normal Functioning Mood.

_____

_____

_____

30—Bad Day Mood.

_____

_____

_____

20—Low-grade Depressed Mood or Dysthymic Disorder.

_____

_____

_____

10—Full Scale Depressed Mood.

_____

_____

_____

0—Unable to Function Mood.

_____

_____

_____

Next steps

Because thinking, feelings, behavior, and moods have been ingrained over many years, it is unlikely that many men will find they can live at a forty-point benchmark most of the time or even for most of each day. It is possible to begin to consciously include mood-lifting behaviors to begin to change the power of the addiction. It is possible to consciously choose forty-point benchmark experiences in order to move out of one's rut.

Pete's story

Pete came for help because he had been found out. Mary, his wife discovered pornographic images and movies on his computer. "Mary told me I either seek help or live in the garage. Not only did I have problems with pornography and masturbation, I worked at least seventy hours a week. I was more married to my job than Mary. I worked long hours, sometimes even weekends. I spent very little time with my teenaged twin boys, Rob and Tom."

Pete, a mortgage broker, quipped, "You have to make hay when the sun shines." Pete had one male friend, a drinking buddy from school. He thought his marriage was acceptable but he did not think that his wife was his best friend. In fact, he said he did not have a best friend. Since he worked so many hours, he told himself, "Sunday morning is my time to sleep and relax." Pete had not been to church for years. The one thing that Pete did have was a healthy stock portfolio. He mused, "Lot of good that will do me when I die of working too hard!" Pete admitted his life was not what he had hoped it would be.

Pete came to therapy scared. Mary had gone back to work when their boys were out of grade school and he knew she made enough money to support herself. He said, "I am afraid Mary is so unhappy she might leave me. Who could blame her? If she leaves me, how will I live? Yes, I have treated her very badly, but I need her."

After several months of therapy, Pete was open to make changes in his life. He explained, "I now understand how healthy and uplifting activities could help to reduce my need to self-medicate my pain. I also know I will be a much happier person if I change my priorities. I need to address my relationships with my family. I need to put them first."

Pete agreed to participate in marriage therapy with Mary. They worked on a marriage plan. He agreed to come home for dinner no later than 6:30 each evening. He and Mary agreed to spend one evening during the week getting to know each other again. They chose to read several books together and to discuss each other's views about what they read. They agreed to do something together each weekend, either a day or evening event. Other changes followed as they became friends.

Pete also addressed his relationship with Rob and Tom. He said, "I am concerned my boys will soon be grown and I will have missed it all. I need to let them know that I take responsibility for my failure to be there for them up to now and begin to 'walk the talk.'"

Pete sat down and talked to his sons. He told them about his addiction to porn and masturbation and the reasons why, as he understood them. The boys already knew, all too well, about Dad's addiction to his work. He asked them to help him repair the damage he had done to their relationship. His sons loved baseball. They agreed to attend minor league games together. Pete made it a point to make time to be with and talk to them. His boys were more than happy to get their dad back.

Pete attended a Twelve Step sexual addiction program and made a good friend with whom he began to share his walk. His friend became his accountability partner.

The next important change Pete made was to repair his relationship with his God. He said, "I asked my family to join me Sunday mornings at church. At first, they did not buy in. I guess they too liked the family habit of sleeping in on Sunday mornings. That's another bad habit I taught them! As I showed by my actions, I was serious about changing my life, Mary joined me at church. One New Year's morning, Rob and Pete said, 'We talked about what kind of New Year's resolution we could make—something meaningful. Dad, we would like to join you and Mom at church each Sunday.'"

Pete made a conscious decision to include activities and other changes that raised his mood functioning to forty. These activities not only raised Pete's mood and reduced his desire to act out, but they made his life much closer to the life he wanted. Chapter 9 addresses some of the changes you may wish to consider to help you experience more forty-point benchmark events.

Note: For those who act out to relieve anxiety, the source of anxiety must be addressed first. For the sexually addicted man steeped in anxiety, a concerted effort to experience forty-point benchmark activities, while needed, will not end acting out. Frequently, medication is helpful to reduce anxiety. Men often find that with medication to reduce anxiety they then can alter their acting out behaviors.

Most of the important things in the world have been accomplished by people who have kept on trying when there seemed to be no hope at all.

Dale Carnegie

Chapter Seven

Is There Hope?

To live without hope is to die. It takes courage to admit you have an unwanted sexual behavior that may or may not be defined as sexual addiction. Labels are not important. If the sexual behaviors in which you are engaged cause you or your family stress, you have a sexual behavior concern. What happens next is up to you.

Facing your unwanted sexual behavior or sexual addiction may be the most difficult task you ever face. What is at stake is the rest of your life! You can continue to live in shame and pain or you can choose to change the dance and enjoy a life of sexual sobriety.

Reinhold Niebuhr's version of the Serenity Prayer captures the philosophy of those journeying on the road to recovery.

Serenity Prayer

Lord, grant me the serenity to accept the things I cannot change;
The courage to change the things I can,
And the Wisdom to know the difference.
Living one day at a time,
Enjoying one moment at a time,
Accepting hardships as the pathways to peace;
Taking, as He did, this sinful world as it is,
Not as I would have it.
Trusting that He will make all things right
If I surrender to His will.
That I may be reasonably happy in this life
And supremely happy with Him forever. Amen.

—Reinhold Niebuhr

Concept of a Journey

Chances are you are not feeling very good about yourself. Most men who finally realize they need to address unwanted sexual behavior, ask themselves several questions:

- Do I really have a problem?

- Is there something wrong with me?

- Am I the only man doing this?

- Am I a bad person?

Others try to convince men that their sexual behavior is not really a problem. "Everyone does it." "It is normal." At the other extreme, our conscience convinces us we are bad, worthless, and evil. With acceptance of, "I am an evil person," we are prone to give up hope. Without hope we live in a dark, scary, and a sad world. With hope, although it may be only a flicker of light far off in the distance, at least there is something to move toward.

Hope from scripture

Scripture, perhaps, is a universal source from which we can gain a clearer understanding of humanity and God's expectation of His people. Sexually addicted men often feel isolated and blame themselves for their shortcomings beyond a realistic comparison to the failings of community and society in general. No one needs to go beyond scripture to see that Christianity was formed on the backs of frail human beings. If God chose the weak to form the backbone of Christianity, then addicted men can take solace that they are not now, nor were they ever alone in their struggle to shed their weaknesses.

Case in point. Christ chose Peter to be the rock upon which He built His church. However, at the time of Christ's greatest need, Peter denied him several times. If there was ever a man who should have given up hope it was Peter. But he didn't. He remained available for God's forgiveness.

The Apostle Paul is not unlike Peter in his behavior. Clearly Paul fully participated in the act of conspiracy to commit murder. He stood by and tended the cloaks of the men who stoned Stephen. He persecuted Christ's followers and yet Christ chose to anoint Paul as His ambassador to bring the Word to the Gentiles.

Christ chose men who were flawed far more than we could ever imagine. These weak men became the pillars of His Church. We, who are sexually addicted, can take comfort. We too can change. We too can change from feeling bad to feeling we are loved.

Let's stay with Paul who tells us:

> To keep me from becoming conceited because of these surpassingly great revelations, there was given me a thorn in my flesh, a messenger of Satan, to torment me. Three times I pleaded with the Lord to take it away from me. But he said to me, "My grace is sufficient for you, for my power is made perfect in weakness." Therefore I will boast all the more gladly about my weaknesses, so that Christ's power may rest on me. That is why, for Christ's sake, I delight in weaknesses, in insults, in hardships, in persecutions, in difficulties. For when I am weak, then I am strong. (2 Corinthians 12:7-10)

Paul does not tell us the specific nature of the thorn in his side. Some scripture scholars speculate that Paul may be referring to some especially persistent and obnoxious opponent. He does not tell us; he only describes his pain. He tells us the thorn was a "messenger of Satan." Paul tells us he asked the Lord to take it away three times and the Lord told Paul, "My grace is sufficient for you, for my power is made perfect in weakness."

Do we dare ask the question, "Did Paul struggle with addiction?" Although there is no way of knowing for sure, some signs may lead to this conclusion. For example:

- Paul tells us the thorn is a "messenger of Satan." Addiction is certainly not a heaven-sent gift. Addiction is a thorn in our side. It is a "messenger of Satan." Could Paul's thorn be his euphemism for addiction?

- Paul tells us he asked the Lord to take his thorn away three times. Would you expect Christ, who personally anointed Paul to be His apostle to the Gentiles, to fail to respond to Paul's plea for the removal of a thorn in his side? Would Christ at least send Paul's messenger of Satan away? No, Paul had to continue to deal with his thorn. Does it sound like addiction?

- Paul tells us in Romans:

> I know that nothing good lives in me, that is, in my sinful nature. For I have the desire to do what is good, but I cannot carry it out. For what I do is not the good I want to do; no, the evil I do not want to do—this I keep on doing. Now if I do what I do not want to do, it is no longer I who do it, but it is sin living in me that does it. (Romans 7: 18-20)

And when Paul tells us, "For I have the desire to do what is good, but I cannot carry it out," (Romans 7: 18) is he not saying he had good intentions but failed? Does he sound like an addicted man who wants to give up his unwanted behavior but fails?

Paul tells us, "For what I do is not the good I want to do; no, the evil I do not want to do—this I keep on doing." (Romans 7: 19) How many times do addicts say "no more" then turn around and repeat their behavior?

Again Paul tells us in Romans:

> . . . [B]ut I see another law at work in the members of my body, waging war against the law of my mind and making me a prisoner of the law of sin at work within my members. What a wretched man I am! Who will rescue me from this body of death? Thanks be to God—through Jesus Christ our Lord! So then, I myself in my mind am a slave to God's law, but in the sinful nature a slave to the law of sin. (Romans 7: 23-25) Could Paul's "waging war against the law of my mind" be temptation toward sexual thinking?

Again Paul talks about his humanness, "making me a prisoner of the law of sin at work within my members. What a wretched man I am!" Paul tells us he feels bad about himself. Addicted men feel bad about themselves, they feel like prisoners, they feel wretched, but they are never outside of God's forgiveness and love.

Paul says, "but in the sinful nature a slave to the law of sin." Is Paul again referring to addiction? Addicted men become slaves to the law of sin; they have difficulty stopping their unwanted sexual behavior.

The lesson we can take away from these hypotheses is, even God's personally anointed apostle struggled with his humanness. He continued to do what he did not want to do. He felt the pain of failure. He had to ask God three times to take away his thorn. He felt "sin at work within my members." His mind and body experienced the pain of sin.

Despite Paul's struggle, he did God's work. If God blessed Paul's struggle, will God not bless your struggle?

Paul found healing and peace. You too can find healing and peace. You, too, can have hope that you can change your behavior.

The change process begins with understanding that the sexual behavior in which you engage is not getting you the satisfaction and the joy of life you desire. Your sexual behavior is simply causing you more pain than the anticipated pleasure. It is time to seek help?

The Lord told Paul, "My grace is sufficient for you, for my power is made perfect in weakness." You too will need to rely on the Lord to help you change the dance, to make a major change in your life.

Changing the dance

You may wonder what your world will look like after you change the "dance." Will all sexual temptations be history? Will you not think about sex anymore? Will you be like a eunuch?

Paul Becker, LPC

The answer probably differs for each person. For some, sexual behavior simply will be rechanneled from unhealthy venues to a relationship supporting arena, that is, to the marriage bed. For others, it will mean abstinence. Because we are sexual beings, it is not likely that you will loose touch with your sexuality. If you are visually stimulated now, it is likely that unchecked visual stimulation will still tempt you. What you do with the temptation, however, will be new.

Most men who are sexually addicted are addicted to sexual behavior on multiple levels.

Sonny's story

Sonny's wife discovered his secret charge account—the account to which he charged his liaisons with prostitutes. In counseling, Sonny revealed that he also frequented massage parlors, engaged in phone sex, enjoyed Internet pornography, and masturbated. He also had an active sexual fantasy world.

Sonny made changes in his acting out behavior. He said, "My marriage will fail unless I give up prostitutes, massage parlors, and phone sex. Let's face it, each of these has a monetary connection and, now that Helen knows, I expect I no longer can hide my expenditure trail."

The fear of future discovery was enough for Sonny to change his most egregious behaviors. After a year of counseling, Sonny was still finding it very difficult to forgo his sexual fantasies and masturbation. However, as time went by, the time span between his slips gradually increased.

Even after Sonny became sexually sober, he found visual temptation to be a continuing problem. Spring was very difficult. One day he shouted, "If I see one more half-naked twenty-year-old, I am going to sue her for confounding the morals of a major!"

Although his comment was cause for a laugh, his expression of exasperation was understandable. Because of his many years of sexual addiction, visual stimulation was likely to remain a source of temptation for Sonny for years to come.

Sonny was able to back down his multiple levels of sexual addiction one layer at a time. Unfortunately, he will never be free of sexual temptation.

Treatment goals

While, through therapy, the addict may achieve sexual sobriety, it will be short-lived unless he makes a significant change in his lifestyle. Long-term and continuing recovery is conditioned upon changing the environment associated with addiction.

According to Carnes (1994), the following are treatment goals:

- Allowing the addict to hear the faulty beliefs of other addicts.

- Breaking through the addict's myths and rules through assignments and permission giving.

- Expanding the addict's options for being nurtured, handling anxiety, and developing a lifestyle congruent with personal values.

- Challenging the addict's family roles and rules.

- Providing information about healthy sexuality. Uncovering multigenerational patterns.

- Giving spiritual assistance.

Addicts' view of the world

Before the sexual addict begins to travel the journey to sexual sobriety, sexual thinking and behavior dominate his world. Visualize a man with a pair of glasses into which a prism has been cut. Everything the man sees is channeled through the prism. The prism is a sexual filter. The prism distorts reality.

What the addict views is conditioned by its sexual connotation. If he sees a woman, he does not see a whole person but a body composed of sexual parts. When he looks at a newspaper, he looks for images to stimulate his sexual thinking. If he goes to the movie, he constantly checks out the actresses for body parts. He is charged up when a sex scene is shown. When he walks into a store, instead of seeing merchandise, he sees women—even mannequins—that feed his sexual fantasies. In other words, the prism turns even innocent images into sexual content. Sexual stimulation is his primary interest.

Is this model relevant to all men who are dealing with unwanted sexual behavior? Only you can say how much your sexual prism dominates your life.

Like most situations, this model for some will be an overstatement, particularly for those who act out because of anxiety. But for many, the model is right on.

World of Addiction

The World of Addiction depicts the mind of a sexual addict. His addiction dominates his life. The time he devotes to other healthy activities and relationships is small compared to the time he devotes to nourishing his addiction.

The Relative
Size of the
Addict's
Sexual World

(90%)

The rest of the addict's world (10%)

New Vision: Recovery

The following are steps the sexual addict may take to shrink the size of his sexual world.

- Forgive self.

- Respect self.

- Seek healthy relationship with God.

- Seek healthy relationships with family and friends.

- Become externally focused.

- Serve others.

- Gain insight and awareness of self and world.

- Foster self care and healthy activities.

- Use interventions and coping mechanisms.

- Live in the present moment.

Note, while the sexual world box shrinks, it does not disappear. Unwanted sexual urges may remain for a lifetime

Family   **Self Care**

                              Marriage

                                                 Career

Leisure Activities

                              Forgive self

Self Respect

                    Relationship with God

Serve others   **Live in the present**

          Friends   **Sexual World**

Coping skills

              Self Awareness

To exist is to change, to change is to mature, to mature is to go on creating oneself endlessly.

Henri Bergson

Chapter Eight

Change the Dance

Life changes

What life changes will help you forgo unwanted sexual behavior? Let's learn from the experience of others.

First a caution is in order here. This book is not a stand-alone solution to your long-term sexual sobriety. Achieving lasting sexual sobriety and healing self are the goals.

This book is intended to help you gain awareness of the world of sexual addiction. It will give you information to process as you ponder what to do next. If you desire to take this book's advice, first seek a counselor trained and skilled in working with sexually addicted men to help you on your journey. Next, find and attend a sexual addiction Twelve Step program. Both are first steps for you. Sexual sobriety is a lifelong journey. Research has found that for most men who deal with unwanted sexual behavior, the journey will likely take five years before a mature level of sobriety is achieved (Carnes, 1992). The journey is for the rest of your life. Likewise, you will also need appropriate support for your entire life.

Why will this book alone not allow you to attain long-term sexual sobriety? In part, the answer is that one solution does not fit all. Yes, for some, following the contents of this book will help gain sexual sobriety for a while but not for the long-term. You are a unique person, and although dealing with unwanted sexual behavior is far from unique, the key for you will be found only after considerable work. Patrick Carnes' (2010) research and considerable clinical experience postulates the completion of thirty specific recovery tasks with a certified sex addiction therapist, individual and group counseling, working the Twelve Step program, and involving the family in the recovery program.

John Bradshaw (1988) proposes three stages of recovery. In the first stage, one addresses the primary addiction. In the second, the addict addresses codependency, getting in touch with feelings, forgiveness, and working on the inner child. In the third stage, he calls for spiritual awakening and empowerment. Both men agree that recovery is a long process, lasting years.

You will need to explore how you became sexually addicted so that you can decide if the model you learned in childhood is the life model you want to follow in adulthood. You will want to examine your acting-out cycle in detail as well as your acting-out rituals. These are only the beginning. You will want to explore what is working in your current life and what is not. Dealing with unwanted sexual behavior is often only the exposed part of the addiction in your life. Dealing only with the behavior and not your underlying needs for love, affirmation, tranquility, respect, etc., is like putting a plastic bandage on an infected wound. Without antibiotics the infection is likely to grow.

Permanently being rid of unwanted sexual behavior involves fundamentally changing important aspects of how you will live the rest of your life.

Awareness Leads to Choices

Counseling, reading other books, and talking to friends, family members, or clergy all begin to raise your awareness of the nature of sexual addiction. Awareness is a beginning point. Awareness leads to choices, which, in turn, lead to changing the dance and changing your life.

An analogy may help: If you think about changing your career path, considerable research and study help you to become more aware of the factors that surround a new career. You will want to know if the career will meet your needs for adventure or security. You will want to know how much education or training will be needed. You will want to know how the change will affect your current and future lifestyle. You will want to be aware of talents that will help you to succeed with a choice to change your career. Changing career paths will likely change the dance—change how you live, your income, friends, commuting patterns, aspirations, and self-esteem.

The same is true when dealing with sexual addiction. Before you can make the choice to change your behavior, you will need to have much more information and understanding about yourself, that is, be much more aware of why you are sexually addicted and what it will mean to change—to change the dance.

Changing the dance—new steps

Recovery means more than giving up an addiction. The "give-up road" often results in the white-knuckle syndrome. You may be prone to failure if you have not addressed the underlying need to act out. Men who use the white-knuckle approach to sobriety fight the same sexual urges over and over. Each time a sexual thought enters their heads they entertain the thought and try to put it out of their heads. Have you ever tried to not think about the thing you are thinking about? Failure is high. The reason is that a high-level commitment has not been made. The white-knuckler plays a game with himself. "Let me try to get this sexual thought out of my head, but not so far out that I can't bring it back later."

The white-knuckler throws away sexually stimulating pornography but keeps a stash. The stash is available for a future time when white-knuckling gets the best of him and relief from the struggle is in order. For example, the stash is sexually stimulating pornography tucked under the mattress or a web link hidden away. The white-knuckler struggles but never fully commits to ending the struggle.

Commitment

The struggle ends when a man is able to make a high-level commitment. A first step toward a high-level commitment is a decision to reject all improper sexual thinking.

Sexual thinking about one's spouse is a blessing, provided such thinking or fantasy does not lead to unwanted sexual behavior.

How does anyone avoid all sexual thinking when random sexual thoughts enter the head without being invited? When a sexual thought enters your mind, through practiced awareness, you will identify the thought as one you do not wish to process within one or two seconds of its beginning. You then will exercise your choice to eliminate the sexual thought, image, or beginning fantasy. One man successfully uses a mantra. He says (aloud when he can), "I do not have the right from God to entertain sexual thoughts!" Another man, who also used a mantra, simply said, "I do not want to go there!" For some men, the repeated use of a mantra helps them achieve their high-level commitment. Their choice is so strong that sexual thinking is banished.

Others, although committed, need more help. Some turn to prayer and others engage in an alternative non-sexual fantasy. One man's favorite time for sexual fantasy was at night, the time right before sleep. He said that sexual fantasy helped to calm him down, but complained, "My sexual thoughts calmed me down except when they excited me to the point that I masturbated." In his case he needed an alternative to sexual thoughts to achieve calm and sleep. He chose an alternative fantasy of playing a round of golf in his head. By the time he completed his alternative fantasy, eighteen holes of golf in his head, he was asleep or onto other acceptable thinking. Some men use other sports fantasies, such as quarterback of a football team, star baseball pitcher, or tennis champion. What is an alternative non-sexual fantasy that you could use as a substitute to sexual thinking?

The key to eliminating unwanted sexual thinking is to recognize what is happening within one or two seconds of the beginning of the sexual thinking process. This takes effort. Often thoughts go on for a longer period of time before cognition that a fantasy has begun. A man has to train himself to become aware of unwanted sexual thinking before the processing begins. Once aware, the choice not to engage in the process further—nada, none, no exception—follows. It cannot be a hit or miss effort. The goal is to end all inappropriate sexually stimulating thoughts, images, and fantasies. The choice to use a mantra reinforces your commitment. Voice it out loud if possible. A mantra is an active reiteration of your commitment. When actively repudiating unwanted behavior, brain chemicals associated with stimulation tend to stabilize. Then use other diversionary tactics that work for you.

For a high-level commitment to have meaning, the effort must begin by eliminating sexual images, fantasies, and sexual thinking. Those who win the battles of the mind find that a reduction in acting out follows. For those who act out because of sheer habit or simply to reduce anxiety, other behavior modifications are needed. In such cases the environmental attributes of the habit need to change. For example, a man who masturbated every night during his shower but did not engage in sexual fantasies found that he had to make shower time uncomfortable. He used music he detested to change his shower time mood and, in time, to change his habit. Men who masturbate to obtain relief from high levels of anxiety found, with the help of a counselor, a need to attack the causes of anxiety in their lives.

Awareness as part of the commitment

Other techniques can be used to defuse the pleasure seeking chemicals that begin to run in the brain. Visual sexual images are not "human" to those who deal with unwanted sexual behavior. Rather, they become objects. The visual sexual images are means of gratification, not opportunities for friendship and relationship building. Taking the object and adding human qualities can change the dynamic of acting out. When one sees a visual sexual image, instead of saying, "I want that." Try replacing "I want that," with, "That person is someone's mother," or "That person is someone's daughter," or "That person could be my sister (or my daughter)." Exploiting someone's mother or daughter, or one's own sister or daughter is not as attractive for most men.

Bill's story

Bill expressed his enjoyment in these words: "Whenever I see a scantily dressed woman, I am off into my fantasy—just she and me. I have been going into my fantasies for so long, how could I give them up? While I tell myself, I don't want to act out, I have grown to like how it makes me feel."

Bill also saw what it was doing to him. He said, "Acting out is the most dishonest thing I do. I like my wife and friends to see me as a good person, but I know that I carry around a secret that, if they knew–well, so much for the good person. When am I going to beat this? When am I going to become the person I want to be? When am I going to put my wife, not my fantasies, first? I have got to try."

Bill learned in counseling that the moment of choice is the instant he becomes aware he is off on one of his fantasies. Awareness must happen before Bill has a choice. Once aware, he can ask himself, "Do I want to go there?"

Bill decided to try sounding his awareness alarm with changing how he viewed scantily clad women. He began to say to himself, "That person could be my sister." It helped but he found he did not fully drop the image. He stored the images in his brain's file cabinet and brought them out as he lay in bed waiting for sleep to come.

Bill talked about his commitment, noting, "I am delaying gratification but I don't seem to be committed to doing away with it. I want to do better. I need to do better. I am sick and tired of the pain. I am sick of being sick."

Bill went back to the drawing board and mapped out a different approach to his awareness alarm. He began individual therapy with a competent sex addiction therapist and he began to attend a Twelve Step program. He found an accountability partner at his church who had struggled with alcohol as a younger man. He talked about his wife. He said he loved her and thought he did not have the right to put fantasizing about other women ahead of his relationship with her. He first dealt with his secrets. With the help of his therapist Bill shared his secret life with his wife. His wife was shocked and hurt but with time she understood the courage it took for Bill to share his shame—his secrets. She understood his desire to make a commitment to put her first.

Bill talked about his approach, noting "I want to make a commitment. I want to stop the pain. To put my fantasies first—myself first—is acting like a selfish child. I don't have a right to do that—it is not fair to Susan or our children. I am going to adopt a new mantra. When I am tempted by a visual sexual image, I will invoke my awareness alarm and I will say to myself, 'I do not have the right to go there.'"

Bill found that it was not an easy commitment. He had been in the habit of entertaining sexual images for a long time. With time, and with the help of his counselor, Twelve Step group, and accountability partner, Bill surrendered himself and began to experience repeated success. He worked on becoming aware of a fantasy and began to exercise his choice, "I do not have the right to go there." He used alternative healthy fantasies, prayer, and other techniques to clear his mind of sexual thoughts.

After about eight months, Bill said, "I really wondered if I could defeat my addiction. It had been part of my life since I was a wet-behind-the-ears kid. My fantasies and masturbation are where I went to deal with my pain. I know that now. An interesting thing happened a few days ago. You know the park on 8th Street? I was driving by and there were a couple of young women lying out in the sun and of course they had much flesh exposed. In the past this would have been more than I could have—you know what I mean? This time, my mantra came into my head—'I do not have the right to go there.' I actually found it easy to continue on my way and leave the girls (someone's daughters) in the park. In fact, I think that it is becoming impossible for me 'to go there.' After having invested eight months of changing my response to environmental temptation, I would be so disappointed in myself if I went back to my old ways. Going there is no longer an option."

Bill found strong reasons for changing his behavior and he used techniques to help clear his mind of offending thoughts. The techniques, by themselves, will not make the difference. But strong commitment along with using techniques made the difference for Bill.

Let's review what Bill did to help himself. He

- found that acting out was causing more pain than pleasure,

- found reasons to change his behavior—his relationship with himself, friends, and most important, Susan, his wife,

- asked a sex addiction therapist to help him and exposed his secrets to the light;

- joined a Twelve Step program,

- asked an accountability partner to help him,

- made a high-level commitment to himself and his loved ones to change his behavior,

- used a mantra each time he came across environmental temptation—"I do not have the right to go there,"

- began to see women, not as objects, but as people who are someone's mother, daughter, etc., and

- worked at his commitment day-by-day until it became part of him.

As time went by Bill and Susan found that their marriage, while better, still had weaknesses. A therapist helped them to understand that they had a codependant relationship. Family therapy helped the family to understand the roles each played and how codependency was an underlying illness that facilitated Bill's sexual addiction.

His individual therapist also taught Bill to change his lifestyle. He programmed in more healthy activities, made new friends, and became closer to his God. He learned that the recovery journey is multifaceted, but it begins with awareness.

Recognize that addiction causes more pain than pleasure

An orgasm is pleasurable. God intended it to be so. However, the period of build-up and orgasm, for most, is a reasonably short period of time. If profound pleasure was not part of acting out, we would certainly find another way of feeling good.

Men trade short periods of pleasure for long periods of shame, guilt, and sadness. Why? One reason is that they do not think of the consequences. They focus on the good feeling. Some men, as they think about the pain-pleasure equation, begin to understand it is far out of balance. The short period of pleasure is not worth the long periods of self-loathing, shame, and guilt. One man said, "I never thought of it that way. It really is dumb what I do to myself."

Men who live in pain for much of their lives often become at ease with that pain. They actually choose pain because it is a comfortable place. It is more comfortable to live in known squalor than to opt for clean, but unknown, quarters. At least they know how pain feels. They fear the unknown because they conclude it will be even more painful. Some call such conclusions, *stinking thinking*. With the help of a therapist, stinking thinking can be disinfected.

As adults we can become aware that living in pain is not getting us what we want in life. Is it time to say, "I don't want to do that any more?"

Address environmental temptation

Visual sexual stimulation is a curse to the sexually addicted man. Even when a man plans to seek sexual sobriety, the media, television, newspaper, and billboard advertisements all sell sex. Advertisers make their wares more attractive by visual sexual stimulation. The Internet is the king of sexual stimulation. In the book, *Every Man's Battle,* the addict is instructed to learn to "bounce your eyes" in the face of visual sexual stimulation (Arterburn, Stoeker and Yorkey, 2000). Bouncing one's eyes, means to shift the eyes from sexually stimulating images upon contact. It is outstanding advice. However, not all men find it possible to bounce their eyes in every situation. Another skill the sexually addicted man can master is understanding that a sexual image is present but reject the processing of the image for stimulation purposes—that is, to drop it.

Let's see how several men reacted to environmental temptation.

Jim's story

Jim was on his way to pick up his young son from a local campus day care center. He said that driving that warm May day through campus set off fire alarms in his brain. He talked about the experience.

"Flesh was everywhere I looked! My intent was not to look but how do you not look when two half-clad students jaywalk right in front you—two students more appropriately dressed for working out in an all women's gym than out on the street. I know it is my problem but, my heavens, I often think like a child in a candy store—so many sweets. I get sick just thinking of sampling all of it."

Jay's story

Jay checks his e-mail each day. A series of recent e-mail messages led him to install a spam blocker. He said: "I have been quite good lately—not going on to the Internet to look at porn. I know that porn leads me to fantasies and fantasies lead me to masturbation. I used to tell myself that I was only going on the Internet to check out the latest pics of Brittany Spears, but I lied to myself. Once there I couldn't stop from checking out a few other sites and I was off to the races. As I said, I have done well over the past few months but last week, I really had a problem. I received several e-mail messages that were provocative, to say the least. I didn't even have to click on them to know that they got my juices running. Right in the e-mail were pictures of young women engaged in—you know what I mean. I wasn't looking for it and surely did not want it but there it was . . ."

Matt's story

Matt likes to watch TV. He says it helps him to relax after a hard day at work. He finds that visual stimulation, particularly images of women with uplifted breasts, begins his sexual ritual. He does not act out if he is not visually stimulated. He said: "I was surfing the channels. I like to watch sports—any kind of sports. Thursday evening, I was home alone and wanted to watch some hockey. Acting out was the farthest thing from my mind. I just wanted to relax and enjoy. I was not prepared for what happened next. I hit a channel (just passing through) and there she was. My reaction was immediate—I could not take my eyes off her. I went down the slippery slope. Why?"

Matt asked a good question: Why? Matt, like many who deal with unwanted sexual stimulation, needs to have a better understanding of what triggers pleasure. With training Matt will be able to develop a different type of alarm. The awareness alarm is triggered when one is visually stimulated and a new thought comes into mind, "I don't want to go there." With self-training this awareness alarm is sounded within the first few seconds of encountering visual stimulation. If Matt allows the awareness alarm to ring before pleasure-seeking chemicals begin to run in his brain, he can choose not to go there. With about six months of repeated success with triggering his awareness alarm at the potential onslaught of visual sexual stimulation, it becomes part of who Matt is. Many find that once the awareness alarm becomes part of their being, it is very difficult to allow visual sexual stimulation to take over.

Address the potential for relapse

Relapse is a reality to a vast majority of sexually addicted men, particularly in the beginning years of their recovery. It is not possible to give a "one fits all" solution because while sex addiction has common characteristics, the specific acting-out triggers and rituals vary among men. A few thoughts are in order:

- During therapy most sex addiction therapists will engage the addict in preparing a "recovery plan" which contains multiple elements that the addict agrees to respect. One of the elements addressed in the plan is relapse prevention. Relapse prevention steps likely include an immediate call to one's accountability partner when the addict finds himself battling the urge to act out.

- If the addict acts out, the recovery plan may include a requirement to immediately document the acting out cycle's four phases and, in particular, the acting-out ritual that led to acting out. The addict is encouraged to examine any possible triggers that began his acting-out cycle.

- The addict is encouraged to share his findings during therapy.

- Far too many times I have heard something like: "I acted out because of (excuse) and I felt bad about myself. However, since I already fell from my sobriety horse, I might as well (binge) for a while." Many men are tempted to act out again once they have fallen and justify themselves through all sorts of "stinking thinking." It is hard for the addict to make a fall a one time event, but recovery is enhanced if it is. Continuing to lie on the ground and continuing to act out is a defeatist attitude. Remember, part of recovery is repatterning the brain away from "greased" neural pathways which facilitate acting out. Binging reestablishes the "greased" neural pathways.

- Advice provided in Chapter 3 warrants repeating. If you fall from your horse named "sobriety" the first subsequent action for you is to get back up and continue your journey. Look at the positive. For example, if you had two weeks of sobriety and succumbed to the urge to act out, it is much more productive to say, "I have a month of sobriety, with a short interruption at week two. After a month or two the fall at week two no longer matters. What matters is, you are continuing to move forward on your recovery journey.

The decision to change is only the beginning. To complete the decision, the sexually addicted man needs to also choose to live a healthier lifestyle. In Chapter 9, we will explore the elements of a changed lifestyle. The journey to sexual sobriety for most men also includes a commitment to spirituality.

The concept of total wellness recognizes that our every thought, word, and behavior affects our greater health and well-being. And we, in turn, are affected not only emotionally but also physically and spiritually.

Greg Anderson

Chapter Nine

Healthy Lifestyle

Changing your lifestyle can diminish your need to act out. When a man chooses to come out of isolation, chooses to improve his relationships with family and friends, chooses to take steps to live at "great to be alive" (forty-point benchmark mood level), chooses to foster a healthy mind and body, and chooses to put God first, he has chosen to change the dance. A healthy lifestyle diminishes the need to self-medicate pain through addiction.

What is a healthy lifestyle?

Making a major change in how you live your life is to engage in a healthier lifestyle. A healthier lifestyle helps to reduce anger, anxiety, and depression and ultimately helps to reduce acting out. If you reduce negativity in your life and thus the need to medicate your pain by acting out, your entire life will be more satisfying. Addressing sexual addiction is not one-dimensional. It means choosing to become a healthier person physically and mentally.

Four basic choices you may wish to consider in choosing to live a healthier lifestyle are: 1) come out of isolation, 2) give up your depressed mood by choosing to take steps to live at "great to be alive," (forty-point benchmark mood level), 3) develop a support system and 4) commit to spirituality.

Coming Out of Isolation

Sexually addicted men live isolated lives. As children, sexually addicted men were often forced to live behind a wall of isolation to survive—out of harm's way of parents who were abusive or did not meet the child's need for affection. As adults they continue to live in their heads. Sexual fantasy and thinking dominate their brain waves. They value their addiction more than their relationships.

Sexually addicted men live in two worlds simultaneously—one visible and one hidden. Although they live in a world others observe, one in which they appear honorable and respected, they always hide their real world, a secret world of sexually acting out. Sexually addicted men build a wall to protect their secrets, a wall of shame. They cry over their loneliness but are afraid to expose their shame. Sexually addicted men are shame-based people.

If you think badly about yourself, it is unlikely you are a loving and gregarious person. You simply lack the self-respect necessary to be loving and gregarious. Because of your shame and guilt, you do not form supportive relationships. It is likely that you do not have a good male friend with whom you share your addiction struggle. It is also likely your marriage is less than what you or your wife desire. The following elements will help you to come out of isolation.

Coming out of isolation by cultivating a strong male friendship

It is vital to cultivate a strong male friendship—a friendship which, in time, will allow you to share the real you, your problems, and your journey. Ideally, you will begin to trust this friend to be your accountability partner. An accountability partner is someone whom you can call to say "the day went well," or "I was tempted to masturbate and I need you to tell me how much God loves me, so that I can let go." The process of developing a strong male relationship takes time. The first step is to identify possible candidates and to initiate an acquaintance. Twelve Step meetings are often a good source of candidates. After all, men in Twelve Step groups understand your pain and you will understand their struggle as well. Another source is a men's group at your church. Many churches have what is called *Celebrate Recovery* groups in which men and women with various addictions come together to seek mutual support.

Interestingly, addicted men generally find it difficult to cultivate a strong male friendship. As children, males are taught to be competitive. Life experiences enforce the stereotype. To show weakness is as bad as it gets for isolated men. For the addicted man, the prospect of forming a strong male relationship means he must let another male into his world of weakness—a very scary thought. Addicted men tend to think they would rather suffer alone in their secret world than willingly show weakness.

The paradox here is that it is precisely the need to share one's weakness that makes the effort to find and make a new male friend so valuable. It is the sharing of the shame that begins to diffuse the underlying need to medicate one's pain by engaging in sexual behavior.

Men who have stepped out of isolation by forming a strong male friendship find the nurturing they never received from their family of origin—an important step on their recovery journey.

Coming out of isolation by improving family relationships

Improving family relationships with parents and siblings is another major step in coming out of isolation. Addicted men often do not have close family relationships. The first reason is that the dysfunctional family-of-origin environment played a strong role in forming the addicted person. It is difficult to love and cherish what hurt them so much. Second, the secret world in which they live is bound by shame on all sides. Taking a risk that Mom, Dad, Sis, or Junior may find out whom Jack really is, a person who engages in lustful behavior and can't stop, is frightening to say the least. Again, it is precisely the need to pierce the shame barrier that begins to defuse the underlying need to medicate pain.

The first step is to engage in a dialogue with family members. The dialogue needs to be deeper than talking about sports or the weather. Since addiction is often a product of childhood experience, a reasonably safe but deeper conversation would be to ask parents and siblings to talk about their memories from childhood. Siblings often have a different perspective of childhood from the addict. Begin the conversation by, "Jim, what was it like for your growing up in our family?" Hearing the perspective of other family members helps to establish a more accurate perception of reality. This is but one suggestion. You will undoubtedly find many more avenues to explore on the way to becoming connected to family in the present time.

Becoming reconnected in a healthy way takes time. Don't be discouraged if your initial efforts yield little. Your isolated way of doing business is what those close to you have witnessed over time. It may take more than one try for them to understand you are trying to change.

Coming out of isolation by improving relationships with a spouse and children

John Bradshaw (1998) discusses how addicts are born in dysfunctional families, and members of dysfunctional families are codependents. Without addressing codependency the family will continue to be dysfunctional. Although addressing the primary sexual addiction is the first order of business, it is essential to address the co-addiction through marital or family therapy.

Improving family relationships with a spouse and children is yet another major step in coming out of isolation, perhaps the most important step.

For the sexual addict, intimacy equates to sex. Sex is an addict's most important need in and out of marriage. It is not difficult then to understand why most couples, where one of the partners is sexually addicted, finds the marriage less than satisfying.

One's spouse is often key to living a more satisfying life. Addicted men must learn to be intimate—and intimacy does not mean sex. Sex needs to be put into a far different perspective. Sex is the dessert, not the nutrition in the meal. Sex is best enjoyed as a product of relationship-based, non-sexual intimacy.

If at least one of the partners is sexually addicted, couples will greatly benefit by changing interaction focus. When the couple is able to say yes to many of the non-sexual intimacy statements below, isolation in the marriage will dissipate.

I know that I have intimacy in my marriage when:

- I consider my partner to be a very good listener.

- My partner understands how I feel.

- We have a good balance of leisure time spent together and separately.

- I look forward to spending time with my partner.

- We find it easy to think of activities to do together.

- I am very satisfied with how we talk to each other.

- We always try to do something nice for each other (without looking for thanks).

- We are creative in how we handle our differences.

- Making joint financial decisions is not difficult.

- We are both equally willing to make adjustments in our relationship.

- I can share feelings and ideas with my partner during disagreements.

- My partner understands my opinions and ideas.

- My partner is my best friend.

- My partner does not try to fix me. We agree it is my job to fix me.

"I have been found out by my wife." This is a statement that led Max and many others like him into therapy. Having been found out is the number one reason men finally seek help for their sexual addiction. A man who comes to the conclusion he needs help and chooses to do so is usually far more motivated to stay the course. In time, Max understood appeasing his wife's anger was not sufficient reason to do the hard work he needed to do on his recovery road. While a self-realization is the best and most productive reason to seek therapy, seeking it due to "getting caught" is better than not seeking it at all.

When a man has been "found out" by his spouse, the marriage is usually in crisis. Although marriage counseling is needed, the timing is often better after the addicted man has been in addiction counseling for at least six months.

Many women who find that their husbands are engaging in sexual activity outside the marriage bed assume that they are married to a pervert and they may have played a role in causing him to be a pervert. Women often try to entice their man back into the marriage bed. Unfortunately, more sex does not solve the addiction.

A wife's common reaction is, "If my husband loved me, he would not go outside the marriage for sex." She sees her man as self-centered, unloving, sex-crazed, dishonest, and untrustworthy. Her trust has been shattered.

Conversely, her husband usually does not see his engagement in sexual activity outside the marriage as having anything to do with his love for his wife or children. A man's mind works differently from that of his wife. This is called *compartmentalization.*

Compartmentalization

Visualize compartmentalization in this way. Picture a man's mind in which are located many boxes. For now let's assume that there are five boxes. Box number one contains his job. In box two is his sexual behavior outside the marriage bed. In box three is his wife and their marriage. In box four are his children. And in box five is the rest of his world, friends, hobbies, etc. A man's mind keeps the boxes separate from each other. He does not focus on how box two, sexual behavior outside the marriage bed, relates to his other boxes. Remember, box two was formed in childhood or teen years, long before the other boxes were formed. Box two became self-contained and part of his secret world at a time when he was unable to choose. Most men hope that box two will go away in marriage, but it simply does not.

Women for the most part do not compartmentalize. In their world, marriage, children, job, etc. are integrated. A woman instantly sees and understands the consequences that box two has on the rest of her world. It is difficult for women to understand men's ability to compartmentalize and often they just can't accept that their man did not see how his acting out sexually would affect her and their family. The women's concept is correct and, with the help of a therapist, the addict will recognize it is time for him to give up the compartmentalized boxes in his head. His sexual behavior ultimately impacts all of his boxes.

Disclosure

Note: Disclosure is best accomplished in the presence of a therapist who is trained to help the addict and, ideally, also competent in providing marital therapy.

Invariably questions about disclosure of your acting-out behavior to your spouse or significant other needs to be addressed. You partner may already know some of your story. Early in the process it is likely she only knows part, for often disclosure happens in phases. She may not know it all and in some circumstances she doesn't need more information.

Addiction counselors are split on whether a man should disclose all of his secrets to his partner. Many therapists believe that a fundamental principle of sexual healing is total honesty and openness in the marriage. They argue, unless disclosure is complete, secrets which remain will distance the partners.

Other therapists believe, while disclosure is the ideal, at times full disclosure opens wounds that will continue for a lifetime. They also believe full disclosure helps the man but inflicts unnecessary pain on his partner. A sexually addicted man may want to disclose his secrets, not for the sake of healing the marriage, but to free himself from the burden of living in a secret world and to purge his conscience. In this type of disclosure the addicted man is disclosing his secrets to reduce his pain, not to establish an honest and intimate relationship.

Your partner's reaction to hearing you disclose your secret world, at a minimum, will cause her hurt and disappointment. However, beyond hurt and disappointment most spouses experience a profound loss of trust and fear for her future and that of the family. It is unlikely you can fully appreciate how your behavior has shattered her dream of a loving marriage. Remember, most sexually addicted men are, for a number of reasons, self centered and inclined to focus on how disclosure will impact on their little world. Husbands often expect their wives to forgive and forget—to compartmentalize.

In a codependent relationship where your partner takes on the role of the parent and feels that it is her responsibility to fix you, information disclosed may become a weapon for her to wield against you. For instance, Nancy badgered Tim for more detail about his affairs. Each time he gave her information she would complain that he was not telling her everything and she could never trust him again. Disclosure in a codependent relationship often continues an unbalanced relationship and may not be wise until codependency is addressed either in individual counseling or later in marital counseling.

Disclosure about events that occurred prior to the marriage relationship can be helpful but only in appropriate detail. Even information about your current acting-out behavior needs to be shared in appropriate detail. Some disclosures may require detail but others may not. Sometimes details cause significant pain for your partner. For example, it is unlikely your partner needs to know precisely how the masseuse provided you with oral sex. The fact that you went to a massage parlor should be sufficient information.

Jane insisted on total detail—of everything that happened. Jane's purpose was not to move on with life once she heard the bad news but to stoke her anger, to keep her anger alive. The more gross the details she heard, the greater her disdain grew for her partner. She insisted on carrying the heavy load of anger when she could have opted for forgiveness which dispels anger. Jane became addicted to her anger and needed fuel to feed her addiction.

Disclosure creates images in the head that may or may not be accurate. Taking information and creating one's own story that distorts reality is unhealthy and creates undue pain. Disclosure can be both a blessing and a curse.

Disclosure is best undertaken in the presence of a trained therapist who can put boundaries around appropriate detail and share insights from years of experience.

An article entitled, *Surviving Disclosure of Infidelity: Results of an International Survey of 164 Recovering Sex Addicts and Partners* concluded:

- Disclosure is often a process, not a one-time event. Even in the absence of a relapse, withholding of information is common.

- Initial disclosure usually is most conducive to healing the relationship in the long run when it includes all the major elements of the acting-out behaviors but avoids the 'gory details.'

- Over half the partners threatened to leave after disclosure, but only one quarter of couples actually separated.

- Half the sex addicts reported one or more major slips or relapses, which necessitated additional decisions about disclosure.

- Neither disclosure nor threats to leave prevented relapse.

- With time, 96% of addicts and 93% of partners came to believe that disclosure had been the right thing.

- Partners need support from professionals and peers during the process of disclosure.

- Honesty is a crucial healing characteristic.

- The most helpful tools for coping with the consequences of sexual addiction are counseling and the Twelve Step programs.

- Disclosure, threats to leave, and relapses are parts of the challenge of treating, and recovering from, addictive disorders." (Schneider, Corley & Irons, 1998).

For women, trust is rebuilt very slowly. In a relationship where each partner is committed to do his or her own healing, information shared about one's journey is treated as "neutral" in contrast to "damning." Accountability information needs to support healing rather than be used as a tool to chastise.

Giving up Depressed Mood

Choose to take steps to live at "great to be alive," (forty-point benchmark mood level)

The sexually addicted man needs to improve his quality of life. He needs to begin to live at a "great to be alive" (forty-point benchmark) mood level rather than a low-level depressed (twenty-point benchmark) mood level so that the pleasure from acting out is substantially lowered relative to lifestyle. When he lives a normal and joy-filled life, the gain from acting out becomes substantially smaller than when he lives in a constant state of a low-grade depressed mood. In other words, when an addict lives at the twenty-point benchmark, acting out yields a thirty-point gain and a temporary release from one's depressed moods. Acting out only warrants a ten-point gain for the addict who has found a way to live his life at the forty-point benchmark. The need to relieve pain begins to go away when a normal and joy-filled life is a daily reality.

Living at forty-point benchmark can mean taking different steps to different people but some common steps include:

- Engaging in healthy recreation. Carve out a period of each week to enjoy life such as biking, walking, playing with one's children, taking one's spouse out to dinner, etc.

- Becoming active in a club or church.

- Engaging your wife or friend in good conversation. Start with fifteen minutes a day and continue to add time. Aim for a good hour of conversation each day.

- Calling one or more friends every day.

- Cultivating a strong male friendship.

- Focusing on what is going right in your life—not what is going wrong.

- Serving others. As part of coming out of isolation, a man can choose to be of service to others. For example, consider serving periodically at a soup kitchen, coaching children's sports, or joining a prison ministry.

Develop a Support Network

Twelve Step programs

Shame is a defining attribute of sexual addiction. It is living in isolation and shame that foster living below the forty-point benchmark. For a man to feel freedom, he has to recognize what caused his addiction, how it took over his life, and how isolated he has become. He also needs to accept the fact that the recovery journey is not a solo adventure. It requires the support of fellow travelers and our Trip Guide, our Higher Power. Twelve Step programs are tried and true. Twelve Step programs address each of these components and more.

Appendix A: Counseling and Support Programs contains more information on Twelve Step programs for sexually addicted men.

An accountability partner

Developing a support network includes being able to call a friend when tempted—a friend who neither judges nor condemns. The sexually addicted man needs an accountability partner. An accountability relationship involves allowing another person to question, challenge, admonish, advise, encourage, and provide input in ways that will help the addict to live his recovery plan.

An accountability partner is a friend who has chosen to love you even when you fail. Although you may want to empower your accountability partner to help you think clearly about your choices, your accountability partner is not your keeper. When you select an accountability partner, look for a person who is well into recovery, a person who has worked his Twelve Steps.

Choose interventions to support your commitment

As part of your support network, include interventions that foster sexual sobriety. Over the years men in counseling have shared techniques or interventions they use to ward off sexual urges. Since every man is unique, you will need to find which of the interventions offered below will help you. Don't be surprised to find you need a unique intervention in your support network.

To make a high-level commitment to end the struggle of sexual thinking and acting out is the ultimate intervention. Much time and effort need to be expended to understand the real difference between white-knuckling and high-level commitment. The interventions you employ before you make a high-level commitment are analogous to plastic bandage strips. They are temporary coverings. They do not cure the wound. The use of interventions alone does not constitute a recovery program.

Paradoxically, once a high-level commitment is made, these same interventions become valuable aids in support of your decision to permanently change your sexual thinking and behavior. As aids they are part of your recovery program.

- Actively participate in Twelve Step and counseling programs.

- Be accountable to yourself—make a conscious choice to eliminate sexual thinking, fantasy, or thoughts.

- Disclose your addiction to an accountability partner or a good male friend. With the aid of a therapist disclose your addiction behavior to your spouse.

- Develop a support network to call in the time of sexual urges. Reach out—call a good male friend or an accountability partner in time of deteriorating mood or when sexual urges begin your acting-out ritual.

- Be aware of your own needs, resentments, stresses, anxiety, and loneliness and how each feeling sets the stage for acting-out sexually. Deal with underlying issues through counseling.

- Medicate anxiety. If feelings of high-level anxiety lead to masturbation to find relief, anti-anxiety medication may help until the source of anxiety is removed. Dealing with high levels of chronic anxiety is toxic both to mental and physical health. (Some medications are addictive and should be taken only under medical supervision. Consult a psychiatrist for a full evaluation and an appropriate prescription.)

- Become aware of your various acting out rituals and learn to recognize when a ritual is beginning. After you experience an acting-out incidence and while the memory is fresh, write down the various steps which led you to act out. Focus on early steps and identify a step at which you became aware you were heading toward a relapse. Preplan an intervention for that stage.

- Become fully aware of the persons, places, feelings, thinking, or things that lead you to act out. Preplan interventions that will diffuse each of these conditions.

- If you are more likely to act out when you are alone, plan ahead not to be alone.

- Become aware of your triggers. Reject them before they happen.

- Put a mantra on your computer, for example, "I will not use this computer to gain access to pornographic material."

- Put a pornography filter on your computer.

- Do not watch TV programs with sexual content. Alternatively, record TV programs you like to watch and fast-forward through sexually disturbing material, ads, or other difficult parts.

- Think through the mantra, "Where am I heading?", when you feel the urge to begin your acting out ritual. Form a mantra that works for you, for example, "I don't have the right to go there!" or "Don't go there," or "I don't have to be a pursuer of my past."

- Just say no! Make a high level commitment to say "no."

- Verbalize cognitive thinking to defuse sexual feelings. In other words, talk out loud to yourself.

- Use an alternative healthy fantasy in place of a sexual fantasy. For example, play fantasy football in your head, play a round of golf in your head, or remember a time when you felt relaxed and enjoyed life.

- Plan more healthy personal time to deal with stress. For example, regular exercise reduces stress. In time of a sexual urge use an immediate exercise intervention such as twenty pushups.

- Intimacy does not equal sex. Learn to practice and enjoy non-sexual intimacy with your spouse. For example, take a walk together, talk about what is important to each of you, and plan other activities that build your relationship. Work to make your spouse your best friend. Spend quality time with your family.

- Understand the factors that foster your choice to live at the forty benchmark and program them into your life.

- Treat yourself to small rewards for not acting out for a set period of time, let's say, a week. One man's self-reward is one hour of shooting pool for every four days of sobriety.

- Understand the degree of pleasure derived from acting out in comparison to the pain of guilt, shame, and time wasted. If the balance is negative, ask yourself why you want to do something that is causing more pain than gain.

- Dispute illogical thinking. If you are lying to yourself or engaging in illogical thinking, admit it and look for truth.

- Learn to bounce your eyes away from sexually titillating images or persons.

- Understand that sexual temptation will continue throughout your life and learn to turn away.

- If you are married, focus on transferring your thinking and your gaze to your wife.

- Instead of seeing a woman as a sex object, see her as someone's mother or daughter. Thank God for making a beautiful woman and let it go.

- Attach a person to a woman or sexual image. See the humanness of the person by focusing on the person's face, eyes, smile, and facial expressions.

- Use a journal to keep in touch with reality—to track moods, lies, triggers, or rituals.

- Work to gain greater awareness of yourself and the world.

- Carry a picture of your family. Take it out when your feel the urge to act out.

- Make environmental adjustments to preclude your acting out ritual—get rid of cable TV or the Internet or choose safe routes.

- Trash stash. *Stash* is sexually stimulating material hidden away in anticipation of a future time of need. Examples include a hidden porno magazine or an Internet URL to connect to a sexually stimulating web page tucked away on your PC.

- Address other addictions—alcohol, drugs, gambling, eating disorders, anger, etc.

- Imagine God's presence in the room when you feel the urge to act out.

- Take a ten minute walk. That is, remove yourself physically from the locus of your sexual urge.

- Carry a motivational verse or scriptural passage to bring you back to reality when you are feeling the urge to act out. Make prayer or other spiritual reading part of your life.

- Play spiritual music to ward off the urge to act out when you are alone.

- Surrender—In the Twelve Step tradition understand and acknowledge it will take both you and the Lord to travel your recovery journey. Ask God's help—understand that the self is powerless.

- Dedicate your home to your God and refrain from acting out there.

- Plan and practice an active spiritual life.

- Have spiritual reading handy in times of sexual urges.

- Learn to forgive yourself.

- If you find yourself living below the forty-point benchmark for weeks at a time, consider going on depression medication combined with individual therapy.

- If you find yourself engaging in outbursts of anger, consider individual therapy.

- If you find your unwanted sexual behavior is continuing, consider individual therapy.

- Make a list of interventions you want to use, post the list where you normally act out, and use it to help yourself.

Note: Each item in the list above either addresses quality of life or actions one can take at the time of an urge to act out. The road to recovery must address both. In the short run, one needs interventions to help to reject a specific temptation. When making your list of interventions include those that address your quality of life and specific temptations.

Planning ahead

Planning activities in advance for periods of depressed mood or interventions for times of temptation have proven to help men. Create and carry two index cards. On one card, list the activities you have preplanned that will take you to the forty-point benchmark. When you recognize your low mood is leading you to act out, review the activities and select one.

On the second card, list interventions you have preplanned to ward off a sexual urge. When tempted to act out, take out the card and select an intervention. These cards will help you to recall activities and interventions at the time of need. It is often difficult to think clearly about alternative activities in time of depressed mood or when you are in the throws of a white-knuckle sexual urge. Planning ahead is an important component of your support network and helps to effectively change the dance.

New behaviors in place of old behaviors

White-knuckling is trying to avert a temptation. When a man thinks of what he is trying to avoid, the process will lead to more temptation. It is impossible not to think of what you are thinking. It is an endless cycle. Instead of white-knuckling, try substituting a new behavior.

Jude's story

Jude found it difficult to stop channel surfing. He said, "As much as I try to white-knuckle through a temptation to search for visual stimulation, I usually fail."

Years ago Jude told his spouse how much he had enjoyed playing pool in his younger days. She encouraged him to purchase a pool table. Instead of watching TV each evening, Jude now engages in a healthy, new behavior, playing pool with his wife. As a bonus they are enjoying each other's company much more.

George's story

George often found it difficult to resist the urge to drive near his favorite places, massage parlors. He said, "It just seems to always happen. I keep telling myself I am not going to go there this time, but I do. Why is it that when I am in my car I get this insatiable urge? What am I going to do?"

George's counselor asked him if changing his acting out ritual would help. George found it difficult to get in touch with how he could change his driving habits. The more they talked, George revealed other parts of his driving ritual. George always played certain oldie-but-goodie music that set the mood for his cruising the massage parlor territory. They agreed to change the music (and the dance). George's new behavior was to listen to spiritual music when he was in his car. He reported that the music—his new behavior—changed his mood and his thinking. It was hard, he said, to listen to spiritual music and seek a massage parlor at the same time.

Both Jude and George put new behaviors in place of old behaviors. New behaviors changed the dance.

Backing off behaviors

Men frequently have more than one form of acting-out behavior. The behaviors also vary in degree of perceived societal acceptance and shame. It is usually easier for the sexually addicted man to end what he considers the most egregious of his behaviors as his first recovery step.

Glen's story

Glen said, "I really enjoy the touch of a woman. I began to go to massage parlors when I was in the service. Overseas, you can find all kinds of services—which used to be really cheap. When I got out and I could afford to treat myself, I had a list of ten or so massage parlors and I made the rounds. I guess at the peak I was spending $1,000 a month. I also liked phone sex. The sound of a sexy woman turned me on. Of course, the Internet and masturbation were also available."

Glen said that he was spending more and more money on sex. He figured he had spent enough money on sex to have bought a twenty-eight-foot boat that sleeps six. He also loved fishing. He wanted to change his acting out behaviors. He said, "You know, after we talked for a few weeks I thought that I could do without the massage parlors and I even cut back on the phone sex."

Glen talked about his reasoning. "Although not spending so much money on sex was a plus, the real motivator for me was fear of being discovered. Can you imagine what it would have done for my career if I was busted in one of those places? I also feared getting a STD. I sure did not want to become an HIV statistic. You just never know."

Glen found it relatively easy to back down from the acting out behaviors that he thought could harm him. He had a much more difficult time giving-up his sexual thinking, the Internet, and masturbation. He said, "Yes, I want to be sexually sober . . . but even after a year of therapy I am still doing it. It seems like it is who I am. The thoughts are always bombarding me. I have a few clean days but I just can't seem to do it."

Glen strongly resisted attending Twelve Step meetings. He thought he was different. He thought he could get in control of his behavior. Glen finally admitted his efforts were not working. He agreed to attend Twelve Step meetings regularly.

"I have not masturbated in several months. My accountability partner is really there for me. I still have another hurdle before I can say that I am well down my recovery journey. I want to end my sexual thinking. It is now time for that to go too."

For some men, backing off behaviors one at a time works. Ideally, foregoing all acting out behaviors from the get-go would be great. For some it takes baby steps—one after another.

Spirituality

Many men find that recovery is only possible after choosing a committed relationship with their God.

Before therapy, sexually addicted men see their God as punishing. Since they feel bad about themselves, why should their God feel any different? An early realization in recovery is to begin to understand that God loves each of us unconditionally, even when we are dealing with the pain of our failings.

While almost everyone has some kind of relationship with God, it is often the relationship with our parents or care givers that shapes our relationship with God.

Dave's story

Dave's early memory of his father was his size and his roar. He said, "My father was a very big man. He was like the giant in Jack and the Bean Stalk. Unfortunately, Dad did not resemble the other famous giant, the Jolly Green Giant. Dad was not jolly. His roar was not happy. It was frightening. He roared often at Mom and us kids. His roar was much louder and more frightening when he was drinking."

Dave's father had a ritual when he punished Dave and his two older brothers. He said, "Dad would take off his belt. He would tell me, 'This is going to hurt me more than it is going to hurt you,' then he would wallop me until I screamed in pain. From the first time I can remember being beaten by Dad, I hated his lie. How could his pain be greater than mine? He did not have welts on his backside. I also remember wondering why Mom would allow Dad to beat me so badly. She knew. So often the beatings were not deserved."

Good moments to remember about Dad were few. Dave explained, "Dad liked to go to the carnival when it came to town. I remember going to the carnival with him and my brother. He began to take us once we were about five years old. In particular, I remember getting my face and hands sticky from eating cotton candy—what a treat it was. One of my older brothers, Ben, was a little league pitcher. He used to practice throwing a ball through a tire hung from a tree—he had great accuracy. He would win several teddy bears until the carnival worker chased us away. Ben once gave me a teddy bear that I kept for many years."

Dave added, "Our family did attend church and I saw Dad pray but I never understood his prayer. He always prayed with his mouth and eyes shut. He never taught me how to pray. Once I asked him about it. His reply was, 'Ask your mother.' I remember thinking that prayer never made Dad a nice person. My older brother introduced me to sex when I was about six. He showed me how to make it feel good. I found those feelings helped me to feel better, particularly after Dad beat me. It was my 'secret time' out behind the shed."

In time, Dave became sexually addicted. He noted, "I grew into a big man like my father. I found my 'secret time' never went away, even after I married."

Dave began counseling when his wife, Julie, told him unless he quit yelling at her and Teddy, their son, she was going to leave and move back with her parents.

Michael, a pastoral counselor, helped Dave explore the linkage between his childhood experiences and his adult life. After several months of counseling he told his counselor about his "secret" time. Dave said, "I remember a session one Thursday evening when I talked about my 'secret' time. I broke down and cried, 'Oh God, where are you when I need you?'"

Michael, his therapist, asked Dave to describe his God. If Dave reached out to God, to whom exactly was Dave reaching out? Who was Dave's God?

He said, "I often try to pray. I close my eyes to pray but words don't come. My image of God is of a very large person with mighty hands and a scowling face. I read in the Bible to fear God. I had that down pat. For years, I thought God was extremely angry at me, you know, about my 'secret' time. I am terrified at the prospect of meeting God when I die."

Michael asked Dave to contrast the image of his father and his God. Dave sat still for several minutes. His face became distorted and he exclaimed, "My God is just like my father!"

Michael said, "Dave, as long as you cry out to an angry God, how do you expect God to help you?" "What do you mean," asked Dave? Michael replied, "Dave, your father was unable to nourish you in the ways you needed in childhood. If your image of God encompasses the same unpleasant characteristics as your father, how can you expect to be nourished by an unnourishing God?"

Michael went on to say, "Dave, you do need to be nourished by God. Let's begin by understanding the incredible love God has for you."

In time, Dave understood God only wants one thing for him—to be his friend. Dave learned God created him and knows his weaknesses. God understands all of mankind's weaknesses. Jesus was human and divine. By being born, Jesus witnessed first-hand human weakness. This was a comforting realization for Dave.

Dave's "secret" time was never a secret from God. God saw what caused Dave's need for "secret" time, and God saw the pain it caused in Dave's life.

God cried with Dave, not at him.

Dave is far from alone. In fact, you may have said to yourself as you read Dave's story, "I know what it is like not to receive the love I needed from my Dad. I know why he turned to his 'secret' time. I know, I know."

When men begin to deal with their unwanted sexual behavior, frequently their image of God resembles the image of their dad. Rarely do they feel the great love God has for them. Most addicted men are like Dave. Their God is angry just as they are angry at themselves and the circumstances that addicted them.

Addicted men have a hole in their soul; that hole needs to be healed.

What does my addiction have to do with God?

Addiction is everything that God is not. God loves. Addiction is painful. God wants to be your rock, your foundation. Addiction is now your foundation—your most important need. God wants your life to be of service to others. Your addiction keeps you bottled up within yourself. God is joy and deserving of praise. Addiction is isolation that keeps you from knowing joy.

Without changing your relationship with God, the journey to sexual sobriety is lonely and painful.

Jason's story

Jason sought help with his addiction because he thought his life was out of control. Jason said, "My sales job brought me big bucks. I spent large sums on prostitution. I traveled and had a girl in every city. I thought I deserved pleasure—I had earned it. If my wife ever found out how much money I spend on my girls, she would sue me for every penny. I am miserable. All I think about are my girls. The defining moment for me was when I chose to spend time with one of my girls rather than respond to a call from one of my most important customers. That bang cost me $25K!"

Jason entered therapy. Within a few months, he gave up his girls. However, Jason pined over how much he missed them. His girls highlighted each counseling session. Jason lived in a state of depression. Although Jason was able to give up his girls, he was far from giving up his sexual addiction. He said, "Pornography and masturbation became my substitutes. I found time to masturbate five or more times each day. I thought I was entitled to a substitute. I realized one day I was spending about a quarter of my day on sex."

After a year in counseling Jason was still masturbating several times a day. No matter what approach was taken, he was unable to change his behavior. During one session he announced he had not acted out for two days. What was the difference? Jason explained, "I heard an evangelist on TV and I became very emotional. I felt like God was talking to me. When I feel in touch with God, I am on an emotional high. I don't feel in touch with God very often. I feel lousy most of the time."

Jason and his counselor explored the similarity between Jason's God-related emotional high and his euphoric feeling at the time of climax. Jason was horrified to realize, but fully agreed, they were similar. They spent several sessions discovering the nature of the healthy relationship God wants with Jason. He began to understand a relationship with God had to be based on his decision to honestly want and to work toward friendship.

Jason said, "As Christmas approached, I made a decision to take my young son, Bret, to church each Sunday. I began to understand that I had to stop acting out or it was very likely I would pass my addictive behavior onto my two sons. Nothing else was working to help me. I can't wait until I am sexually sober, to ask God to come into my life. Even when it was not convenient, I continued to take Bret to church each Sunday. Bret looked forward to Sunday morning—time alone with me. I want the relationship between me and Bret to be different from the one between my dad and me."

About a month later, Jason came to his session with a smile on his face. He said, "I have been sexually sober for a week. I began to think differently once I made the decision to change my relationship with God. My view of life changed. Something is different now. Life is more than meeting my needs. I feel closer to my boys and my wife. My wife said I am different."

Jason kept his commitment to attend church with Bret. He began to explore other aspects of his relationship with God. He has come out of isolation and is trying to help family members through difficult times. He is sharing his extra money with family members who desperately need a helping hand.

Jason periodically talks about missing his old lifestyle but his laments grow fewer over time. He said he no longer could turn his back on his family and God. He said his investment is far too precious to him. "I simply can't go back to acting out."

Nothing in counseling worked for Jason until he made the decision to turn to God.

Committed and genuine relationship with God

In your life of addiction, sexual pleasure is your commitment. You do what it takes to repeat the experience over and over. The only problem is, it never makes you feel good for longer than a short period of time, generally the time it takes you to complete your acting out ritual. It is a search for the Holy Grail—a search with no end, no Holy Grail.

In an article, *What Does it Take for a Family to Recover,?* Earl Henslin (1991), describes the committed and genuine relationship with God this way:

> No authentic and long-lasting change occurs without God's help and the work of the Holy Spirit in a person's life. A committed and genuine spirituality is an essential foundation for recovery. By *genuine* I mean spirituality that is biblically based and authentic—a real experience with God, not simply going through the motions. By *committed* I mean a relationship with God in which you dedicate yourself to godly living as far as it lies in your power . . . By *committed* and *genuine* I do not mean a perfect spirituality (whatever that is). God begins with us where we are.

Engaging in a committed and genuine relationship with Christ is paramount to finding the true Holy Grail. After the pain and misery of addiction, embrace Christ as the Holy Grail.

Surrender

In Jason's story, life began to change when he found his God was a God of love, not a reflection of childhood experiences. He needed help; he could not recover on his own. Twelve Step programs call this experience surrender. In Sexaholics Anonymous (1989), surrender is characterized as a change in attitude.

> [F]or us surrender is the change in attitude of the inner person that makes life possible. It is the great beginning, the insignia and watchword of our program. And no amount of knowledge about surrender can make it a fact until we simply give up, let go, and let God in. When we surrender our "freedom," we become truly free.

Surrender is a spiritual experience. It is a very calming experience. The addict has tried time and again to "gain control" over his acting out only to experience slip after slip. Addict control simply does not work. Working a Twelve Step program, surrendering control to God, and relying on others to guide you does work.

Concluding thoughts

In this book, you have explored the steps to begin a recovery program from sex addiction. You now know that you cannot successfully make this journey on your own. You will need the support of God, a counselor, an accountability partner, family members, friends, and your spouse. Stepping out of isolation can be terrifying, but like many men before you, it is possible to discover the healing and hope offered through recovery.

Virtually every sexually addicted man with whom I have worked found his relationship with God damaged by his sexual behavior. It was not God who backed away from the relationship. It is the shame of our behavior that causes distancing. I eventually learned that God loves me no matter what I've done in the past. God even loved me when I was responding to sexual urges.

God loves you and he always will. I ask you to accept this premise as the first milestone in your recovery path. May you come to know that a loving God is available to guide you on your path.

Appendix A

Counseling and Support Programs

How Do I Get Help?

Help for the sexually addicted man comes in many forms. In this section you will find many venues for help including counseling and Twelve Step programs. All of the material provided has been downloaded from public Web sites.

Individual Counseling

Society for the Advancement of Sexual Health (SASH) provides a Web site reference section where interested men can search for the names of sex addiction counselors in specific locations. The Web site is http://www.sash.net/.

The American Association of Pastoral Counselors also provides a geographic reference service. Note that not all pastoral counselors are trained to provide sexual addiction counseling. The Web site is: http://www.aapc.org/.

When the words sexual addiction counseling were entered into Google's search engine, more than a million hits were returned. Modify your search to sex addiction counselor followed by your city and state.

When searching for a counselor it is critical to find a competent person with whom you are comfortable. Ask if the counselor provides a consultation session. If so, in the session talk about the counseling methods the counselor uses. During that time you can assess your compatibility with the counselor.

Twelve Step programs

The following is an inventory of the major Twelve Step and related programs that are available to those who desire recovery from sexual addiction. The list contains the name, link to an Internet Web page, and a brief description of the purpose of each organization. This book endorses Twelve Step programs but does not endorse a specific Twelve Step program. It is for you to decide which Twelve Step program best fits your needs. You may wish to try more than one program.

Twelve Step programs for the addict

Christians in Recovery

The Web site is http://christians-in-recovery.org/wp/

Christians in Recovery (CIR) is a group of recovering Christians dedicated to mutual sharing of faith, strength and hope as we live each day in recovery. We work to regain and maintain balance and order in our lives through active discussion of the 12 Steps, the Bible, and experiences in our own recovery from abuse, family dysfunction, depression, anxiety, grief, relationships and/ or addictions of alcohol, drugs, food, pornography, sexual addiction, etc.

Sex Addicts Anonymous

The Web site is http://www.sexaa.org/.

Sex Addicts Anonymous is a fellowship of men and women who share their experience, strength and hope with each other so they may overcome their sexual addiction and help others recover from sexual addiction and dependency. Membership is open to all who share a desire to stop addictive sexual behavior. There is no other requirement.

Our common goals are to become sexually healthy and to help other sex addicts achieve freedom from compulsive sexual behavior. SAA is supported through voluntary contributions from members. We are not affiliated with any other Twelve Step programs, nor are we a part of any other organization. We do not support, endorse, or oppose outside causes or issues.

Sex Addicts Anonymous is a spiritual program based on the principles and traditions of Alcoholics Anonymous. We are grateful to A.A. for this gift which makes our recovery possible.

Sexaholics Anonymous

The Web site is http://www.sa.org/.

Sexaholics Anonymous is a fellowship of men and women who share their experience, strength, and hope with each other that they may solve their common problem and help others to recover.

The only requirement for membership is a desire to stop lusting and become sexually sober. There are no dues or fees for SA membership; we are self-supporting through our own contributions.

SA is not allied with any sect, denomination, politics, organization, or institution; does not wish to engage in any controversy; neither endorses nor opposes any causes.

Our primary purpose is to stay sexually sober and help others to achieve sexual sobriety. Sexaholics Anonymous is a recovery program based on the principles of Alcoholics Anonymous.

Sexual Compulsives Anonymous

The Web site is http://www.sca-recovery.org/.

Sexual Compulsives Anonymous is a fellowship of men and women who share their experience, strength and hope with each other, that they may solve their common problem and help others to recover from sexual compulsion.

SCA is a Twelve Step fellowship, inclusive of all sexual orientations, open to anyone with a desire to recover from sexual compulsion. We are not group therapy, but a spiritual program that provides a safe environment for working on problems of sexual addiction and sexual sobriety.

We believe we are not meant to repress our God-given sexuality, but to learn how to express it in ways that will not make unreasonable demands on our time and energy, place us in legal jeopardy, or endanger our mental, physical or spiritual health. Members are encouraged to develop a sexual recovery plan, defining sexual sobriety for themselves.

There are no requirements for admission to our meetings: anyone having difficulties with sexual compulsion is welcome. The only requirement for membership is a desire to stop having compulsive sex. There are no dues or fees for SCA membership; we are self-supporting through our own contributions. SCA is not allied with any sect, denomination, politics, organization, or institution; does not wish to engage in any controversy; neither endorses nor opposes any causes.

Our primary purpose is to stay sexually sober and to help others to achieve sexual sobriety.

Sex and Love Addicts Anonymous

The Web site is http://www.slaafws.org/.

Sex and Love Addicts Anonymous is a Twelve Step—Twelve Tradition oriented fellowship based on the model pioneered by Alcoholics Anonymous.

One of the resources we draw on is our willingness to stop acting out in our own personal bottom line addictive behavior on a daily basis. In addition, members reach out to others in the fellowship, practice the Twelve Steps and Twelve Traditions of S.L.A.A. and seek a relationship with a higher power to counter the destructive consequences of one or more addictive behaviors related to sex addiction, love addiction, dependency on romantic attachments, emotional dependency, and sexual, social and emotional anorexia.

We find a common denominator in our obsessive, compulsive patterns which renders any personal differences of sexual or gender orientation irrelevant.

Sexual Recovery Anonymous

The Web site is http://www.sexualrecovery.org/.

Sexual Recovery Anonymous (SRA) is a fellowship of men and women who share their experience, strength and hope with each other that they may solve their common problem and help others to recover.

The only requirement for membership is a desire to stop compulsive sexual behavior. There are no dues or fees for SRA membership; we are self-supporting through our own contributions. SRA is not allied with any sect, denomination, politics, organization, or institution; does not wish to engage in any controversy; neither endorses nor opposes any causes.

Our primary purpose is to stay sexually sober and help others achieve sobriety. Sobriety is the release from all compulsive and destructive sexual behaviors. We have found through our experience that sobriety includes freedom from masturbation and sex outside a mutually committed relationship.

We believe that spirituality and self-love are antidotes to the addiction. We are walking towards a healthy sexuality.

Survivors of Incest Anonymous (SIA)

The Web site is http://www.siawso.org/.

Survivors of Incest Anonymous (SIA) is a self-help group of women and men, 18 years or older, who are guided by a set of 12 Suggested Steps and 12 Traditions, along with some slogans and the Serenity Prayer. There are no dues or fees. Everything that is said here, in the group meeting or member to member, must be held in strict confidence. We do not have any professional therapist working in our group. SIA is not a replacement for therapy or any other professional service when needed. The only requirement for membership is that you are a victim of child sexual abuse, and you are not abusing any child. We define incest very broadly as a sexual experience by a family member or by an extended family member that damaged the child. "Extended family" may include an aunt, uncle, in-law, step-parent, cousin, friend of the family, teacher, coach, another child, clergy or anyone that you were led to trust. We believe we were affected by the abuse whether it occurred once or many times since the damage is incurred immediately.

We learn in SIA not to deny, that we did not imagine the incest, nor was it our fault in any way. The abuser will go to any length to shift the responsibility to the defenseless child, often accusing the child of being seductive. We had healthy, natural needs for love, attention and acceptance, and we often paid high prices to get those needs met, but we did not seduce our abuser. Physical coercion is rarely necessary with a child since the child is already intimidated. The more gentle the assault, the more guilt the victim inappropriately carries. We also learn not to accept any responsibility for the assaults even if these occurred over a prolonged period of time. Some of us are still being sexually assaulted.

In SIA we share our experiences and common feelings. We realize that we thought we had to protect our caretakers from this horrible secret, as if they were not participants. We felt alienated from the non-abusive family members. Often, greater anger is directed toward them since it is safer to get angry at people we perceive to be powerless. We became caretakers in order to maintain an image of a nurturing family. Our feelings of betrayal by our families are immeasurable. We need to mourn the death of the ideal family that many of us created in our own imaginations.

In dealing with this pain, it feels as if we are pulling the scab off a wound that never healed properly, AND IT HURTS. However, it is easier to cry when we have friends who are not afraid of our tears. We CAN be comforted—that is why we are here. Our pain is no longer in vain. We will never forget, but we can, in time, end the regretting that accompanies destructive remembering. We can learn, One Day at a Time, that we are incest SURVIVORS, rather than incest victims.

Incest Survivors Anonymous (ISA)

The Web site is http://www.lafn.org/medical/isa/home.html.

Incest Survivors Anonymous (ISA) is:

- A spiritual program.

- A Twelve Step and Twelve Tradition program for incest survivors and prosurvivors. Prosurvivor is someone who loves, believes, and supports the survivor in their recovery from incest, such as a family member, spouse, friend.

- An anonymous fellowship.

- Self-help, peer-help.

- Unconditional love.

- For men, women, teens.

Recovering Couples Anonymous(RCA)

The Web site is http://www.recovering-couples.org/.

> Recovering Couples Anonymous (RCA) is a 12-Step Fellowship founded in the Autumn of 1988. There are groups throughout the United States, as well as worldwide. Although there is no organizational affiliation with Alcoholics Anonymous, The 12 Steps, 12 Traditions and Principles are adapted from AA.

> The primary purpose of RCA is to help couples find freedom from dysfunctional patterns in relationships. By using the tools of the program, we take individual responsibility for the well-being of the relationship, build new joy, and find intimacy with each other.

> We are couples committed to restoring healthy communication, caring and greater intimacy to our relationships. We suffer from many addictions and co-addictions; some identified and some not, some treated and some not. We also come from different levels of brokenness. Many of us have been separated or near divorce. Some of us are new in our relationships and seek to build intimacy as we grow together as couples.

Twelve Step programs for the spouse or significant other

Codependents of Sexual Addiction

The Web site is http://www.cosa-recovery.org/.

> Codependents of Sexual Addiction (COSA) is a recovery program for men and women whose lives have been affected by compulsive sexual behavior. In COSA, we find hope whether or not there is a sexually addicted person currently in our lives. With the humble act of reaching out, we begin the process of recovery.

> The COSA recovery program has been adapted from the Twelve Steps and Twelve Traditions of Alcoholics Anonymous and Al-Anon. It is a program for our spiritual development, no matter what our religious beliefs. As we meet to share our experience, strength and hope while working the twelve steps, we

grow stronger in spirit. We begin to lead our lives more serenely and in deeper fulfillment, little by little, one day at a time. Only in this way can we be of help to others.

COSA is open to anyone whose life has been affected by compulsive sexual behavior. Although there are no dues or fees for membership, most groups pass a basket for contributions since COSA is entirely self-supporting and declines outside donations.

S-Anon Family Groups

The Web site is http://www.sanon.org/.

The S-Anon Family Groups are a fellowship of the relatives and friends of sexually addicted people who share their experience, strength and hope in order to solve their common problems. Our program of recovery is adapted from Alcoholics Anonymous and is based on the Twelve Steps and the Twelve Traditions of Alcoholics Anonymous. S-Anon's Twelve Concepts of Service provide guidance in serving each other in our business matters. There are no dues or fees for S-Anon membership; we are self-supporting through our own contributions.

S-Anon is not allied with any sect, denomination, politics, organization or institution; it does not wish to engage in any controversy; nor does it endorse or oppose any causes. Our primary purpose is to recover from the effects upon us of another person's sexaholism and to help the families and friends of sexaholics. We do this by applying the Twelve Steps of S-Anon to our lives and by welcoming and giving comfort to families of sexaholics.

Appendix B

Suggest Readings

Note: Book descriptions originated from book-seller Web sites and were edited for this appendix.

Books by Dr. Patrick Carnes

Carnes, P. (1994). Contrary To Love: Helping the Sexual Addict. Center City, MN: Hazelden.

> This book provides counseling professionals with a resource for understanding and helping sexual addicts. Subjects include stages and progression of the illness, family structures, boundaries, assessment, and intervention. The book presents a Sexual Addiction Screening test, useful to therapists and addicts alike. The book is a sequel to Out of the Shadows.

Carnes, P. (1992). Don't Call It Love: Recovering From Sexual Addiction.
New York: Bantam.

> This book describes sexual addiction and its characteristics based on the testimony of more than one thousand recovering sexual addicts. It is the first major scientific study of the disorder. It includes the findings of Dr. Carnes' research with recovering addicts as well as advice from the addicts and coaddicts themselves as they work to overcome their compulsive behavior.

Carnes, P. (1994). A Gentle Path Through the Twelve Steps: A Guidebook for all People in the Process of Recovery. (Rev. Ed.). Center City, MN: Hazelden.

> This workbook provides a unique set of structured forms and practical exercises to help recovering people integrate the Twelve Steps into all aspects of their lives. It is the first workbook on the Twelve Steps specifically designed with sex addicts and coaddicts in mind.

Carnes, P. (1997). Sexual Anorexia: Overcoming Sexual Self-Hatred. Center City, MN: Hazelden.

> This book is a first-time examination of sexual anorexia: the extreme fear of sexual intimacy and obsessive avoidance of sex. It examines its causes,

then describes concrete tasks and plans for exploring intimacy and restoring healthy sexuality.

Carnes, P. (1997). The Betrayal Bond: Breaking Free of Exploitive Relationships. Deerfield Beach, FL: Health Communications Inc.

> This book presents an in-depth study of exploitive relationships: why they form, who is most susceptible, and how they become so powerful. It explains to readers how to recognize when traumatic bonding has occurred and provides a checklist so they can examine their own relationships. Included are steps readers can take to safely extricate themselves or their loved ones from these situations.

Carnes, P. & Harkin, M. (2010). Facing the Shadow: Starting Sexual and Relationship Recovery. (2nd ed.). Carefree, AZ: Gentle Path Press.

> This workbook is designed as a companion to Out of the Shadows, Don't Call It Love, and Sexual Anorexia. It includes exercises to help work through such subjects as denial, understanding the addictive cycle, and identifying compulsive behaviors.

Carnes, P. (2001). Out of the Shadows: Understanding Sexual Addiction (Rev. 3rd ed.). Center City, MN: Hazelden.

> This book, the first to describe sexual addiction, is the standard for recognizing and overcoming this destructive behavior. It outlines how to identify a sexual addict, recognize the way others may unwittingly become complicit or codependent, and change the patterns that support the addiction.

Carnes, P., Lasser, D., & Lasser, M. (1999). Open Hearts: Renewing Relationships with Recovery, Romance and Reality. Carefree, AZ: Gentle Path Press.

> This book will guide the reader along a pathway of self-assessment, discovery, and fulfillment. Proven techniques from Recovering Couples Anonymous help couples overcome anger, resentment, and dysfunctional patterns, thus allowing them to enjoy the intimate, fulfilling relationship they long for. It is a book a couple does together. It takes techniques Carnes and Laaser developed in their psychotherapy practices and weaves them into a series of individual and joint exercises. It looks at tough issues: shame, anger, money, betrayal, sex, parenting. It encourages fun like drawing up a family motto, expressing spirituality together, and taking gentleness breaks.

Carnes, P., Delmonico, D. & Griffin, E. (2001). In the Shadows of the Net: Breaking Free of Compulsive Online Sexual Behavior. (2nd Ed.). Center City, MN: Hazelden.

> This book explains how the anonymity of online access, the ability of people to use their computers in private, and the powerful rationalization that virtual

interactions are not "real" can combine to entice people to spend hours online, sacrificing real relationships and increasing their sense of loneliness. The book provides a Internet Screening Test to help people decide if they have a problem with their use of sexual material on the Internet.

Carnes, P., & Adams, K. (2002). The Clinical Management of Sex Addiction. New York, NY: Brunner-Routledge.

This is the first comprehensive volume of the clinical management of sex addiction. Collecting the work of twenty-eight leaders in this emerging field, the editors provide a long-needed primary text about how to approach treatment with these challenging patients. The book serves as an introduction for professionals new to the field as well as serving as a useful reference tool. The contributors are pioneers of addiction medicine and sex therapy.

Carnes, P. (2009). Recovery Zone, Volume 1: Making Changes that Last, The Internal Tasks. Carefree, AZ: Gentle Path Press.

This workbook notes that recovery from addiction is a work in progress and that many things must change simultaneously for recovery to work. The book shares strategies for maintaining and nurturing recovery, in the early days and beyond.

Other Readings

Arterburn, S., Stoeker, F., & Yorkey, M. (2000). Every Man's Battle: Winning the War on Sexual Temptation One Victory at a Time. Colorado Springs, CO: WaterBrook Press.

This book describes the challenge every man faces . . . the fight every man can win . . . sexual temptation. From the television to the Internet, print media to videos, men are constantly faced with the assault of sensual images. The book denies the perception men are unable to control their thought lives and roving eyes. The book shares the stories of men who have escaped the trap of sexual immorality and presents a practical, detailed plan for any man who desires sexual purity-perfect for men who have fallen in the past, those who want to remain strong today, and all who want to overcome temptation in the future. It includes a section for women, designed to help them understand and support the men they love.

Arterburn, S., Stoeker, F., & Yorkey, M. (2002). Every Man's Battle Workbook: The Path to Sexual Integrity Starts Here. Colorado Springs, CO: WaterBrook Press.

This book is a practical guide for individuals and men's groups designed to help men win the war on sexual temptation. It is a companion workbook to Every Man's Battle.

Becker, P. (2012). Why Is My Partner Sexually Addicted? Insight Women Need. Bloomington, IN: AuthorHouse.

> A woman rarely has a need to understand the origin and consequences of sexual addiction until someone close is found to exhibit sex addiction behavior. Each of the chapters in this book reveal aspects of sexual addiction, all to help a women understand her partner's betrayal and to enable her to decide how she will live her life in the future. If you are confounded by the discovery of your partner's aberrant sexual behavior and need to understand why this is happening to you and your family, this book is for you!

Black, C. (2002). It Will Never Happen to Me: Growing Up With Addiction As Youngsters, Adolescents, Adults. (2nd ed.). Center City, MN: Hazelden.

> This book identifies common issues faced by children who grew up in alcoholic families—shame, neglect, unreasonable role expectations, and physical abuse. Using narratives and profiles, Black describes survival techniques characteristic of children raised in alcoholic families, including the unspoken laws of don't talk, don't trust, and don't feel.

Black, C. (2009). Deceived: Facing Sexual Betrayal Lies and Secrets. Center City, MN: Hazelden.

> No matter the 'drug' of choice, men who act out sexually leave their partners reeling in fear, rage, incredible shame, and isolation. Deceived was written expressly to help women better understand what is happening in their lives, garner validation for their experiences, and find a path that offers clarity, direction, and voice.

Black, C. (2000). A Hole in the Sidewalk: The Recovering Person's Guide to Relapse Prevention. Center City, MN: Hazelden.

> The journey along the road to recovery may be a glorious and fulfilling adventure, but there are dangers and pitfalls along the way. The person recovering from any addiction needs to be aware of the hazards that lead to relapse. A Hole in the Sidewalk points out ways to avoid the holes; as one travels the path of recovery.

Bradshaw, J. (1988). Bradshaw on: The Family. Deerfield Beach, FL: Health Communications.

> This book focuses on the dynamics of the family, how the rules and attitudes learned while growing up become encoded within each family member. It guides the reader out of dysfunction to wholeness and teaches bad beginnings can be remedied.

Carnes, S. (Ed.). (2011). Mending a Shattered Heart: A Guide for Partners of Sex Addicts 2nd ed. Carefree, AZ: Gentle Path Press.

This book is for the spouse who needs an answer to the question: Where do I go from here? Many discover their loved one, the one person that they are supposed to trust, has been living a life of lies and deceit because they suffer from sex addiction.

Cooper, A. (Ed.). (2001). Sex and the Internet: A Guide for Clinicians. New York, NY: Brunner-Routledge.

Sex and the Internet is the first professional book on Internet sexuality. This book is a clinician's guide that addresses Internet sexuality by both informing and providing practical and concrete suggestions and directions. The book is compilation of contributions by international experts in the field of sexuality including Patrick Carnes.

Corley, D., & Schneider, J. (2002). Disclosing Secrets: When, to Whom and How Much and to Reveal. Carefree, AZ: Gentle Path Press.

This book is a guide to revealing sexual addiction secrets to one's spouse and others. The book takes the reader through the painful process of revealing addiction related secrets . . . what, where, when to tell and who to involve.

Crow, G., Earle R., & Osborn, K. (1989). Lonely All the Time: Recognizing, Understanding and Overcoming Sex Addiction, for Addicts and Codependents. New York, NY: Pocket Books (Div. Of Simon & Schuster).

This book is a comprehensive, practical approach to recovery for the addict. It explains what sex addiction is and how to recover from sex addiction. The book explores the causes and symptoms of sex addiction. It also includes a practical approach to recovery for the addict and family.

Gordon, J. R., & Marlat, G. A. (Eds.). (1985). Relapse Prevention: Maintenance Strategies in the Treatment of Addictive Behaviors. New York, NY: Guilford Publications.

This book analyzes factors that may lead to relapse and offers practical techniques for maintaining treatment gains.

Hendrix, H. (2001). Getting the Love You Want: A Guide for Couples (Rep. ed.). New York, NY: Owl Books.

This book presents relationship skills to help couples replace confrontation and criticism with a healing process of mutual growth and support. It describes the techniques of Imago Relationship Therapy, which combines a number of disciplines—including the behavioral sciences, depth psychology, cognitive therapy, and Gestalt therapy, among others—to create a program to resolve conflict and renew communication and passion.

Hope and Recovery: A Twelve Step Guide for Healing From Compulsive Sexual Behavior. (1987). Minneapolis, MI: CompCare Publishers.

This was one of the first books to comprehensively describe the application of the Twelve Steps of Alcoholics Anonymous to sexual addiction and compulsivity. It also includes a wide range of personal stories in which recovering sexual addicts share their experience, strength, and hope.

Kasl, C. D. (2002). Many Roads, One Journey: Moving Beyond the Twelve Steps. Saint Helens, OR: Perennial Press.

This book, from the author of Women, Sex, and Addiction, is a timely and controversial second look at Twelve Step programs. It is intended to help readers draw on the steps' underlying wisdom and adapting them to their own experiences, beliefs, and sources of strength.

Laaser, M. (2004). Healing the Wounds of Sexual Addiction. Grand Rapids, MI: Zondervan Publishing Company.

This book is written by a former sex addict. It offers help and hope for regaining and maintaining sexual integrity, self-control, and wholesome, biblical sexuality.

Maltz, W. (2001). The Sexual Healing Journey: A Guide for Survivors of Sexual Abuse (Rev. Ed.). New York, NY: Harper Perennial.

This comprehensive guide will help survivors of sexual abuse improve their relationships and discover the joys of sexual intimacy. Maltz takes survivors step-by-step through the recovery process using groundbreaking exercises and techniques.

Maltz, W. & Malty, L. (2009). The Porn Trap: The Essential Guide to Overcoming Problems Caused by Pornography. (Reprint Ed.) New York, NY: William Morrow Paperbacks.

This book sheds new light on the compelling nature and destructive power of today's instantly available pornography. Weaving together poignant real-life stories with innovative exercises, checklists, and expert advice, this groundbreaking resource provides a comprehensive program for understanding and healing porn addiction and other serious consequences of porn use.

Mellody, P. (1989).Facing Codependence: What It Is, Where It Comes from, How It Sabotages Our Lives. New Your, NY: Harper & Row.

> The author creates a framework for identifying codependent thinking, emotions and behavior and provides an effective approach to recovery. The book sets forth five primary adult symptoms of this crippling condition, then traces their origin to emotional, spiritual, intellectual, physical and sexual abuses that occur in childhood. Central to the approach is the concept that the codependent adult's injured inner child needs healing. Recovery from codependence, therefore, involves clearing up the toxic emotions left over from these painful childhood experiences.

Milkman, H., & Sunderwirth, S. (1998). Craving for Ecstasy: How Our Passions Become Addictions and What We Can Do About Them (Rep ed.). San Francisco, CA: Jossey-Bass.

> The book describe the variety of addictive ways individuals lose control of their lives while striving for pleasure and escape. Addictive behavior goes beyond the compulsive use of drugs and alcohol. It is possible to become addicted to what may seem a harmless pleasure such as sex, jogging, watching television, and eating. This book explains the biology, chemistry, and psychology of the universal desire for pleasure and escape. For example, it reveals how the brain produces "mind-altering" substances and what the skydiver has in common with the heroin addict. With the use of a self-assessment test and an a guide for treatment, the book shows what steps one can take to regain control of one's life.

Schaumburg, H. (1997). False Intimacy: Understanding the Struggle of Sexual Addiction (Rev. ed.). Colorado Springs, CO: Navpress Publishing Group.

> This book, set in a Christian context, examines the roots behind destructive sexual behaviors and offers realistic direction to those whose lives or ministries have been impacted by sexual addiction.

Schneider, J. (2001). Back from Betrayal: Recovering from His Affairs (2nd ed.). Recovery Resources Press.

> This book provides practical help for women involved with sex addicted men. The second edition is expanded and updated, with a new chapter for men whose partner is a sex addict, and another new chapter on living with a cybersex addict.

Schneider, B., & Schneider, J. (2004). Sex Lies and Forgiveness: Couples Speaking Out on Healing from Sex Addiction (3rd ed.). Recovery Resources Press.

> In this book, 88 couples talk about how they have coped with the problem of addictive sexual behavior.

Schneider, J. & Weiss, R. (2001) Cybersex Exposed: Simple Fantasy or Obsession? Center City, MN: Hazelden Publishing & Educational Services.

Examining the negative consequences of Internet sex addiction on health, career, intimacy and family relationships, this guide provides a test to help readers evaluate their own behavior. The guide also discusses the negative impact of cybersex on partners and presents stories of recovery.

Steffens, B. (2009). Your Sexually Addicted Spouse: How Partners Can Cope and Heal Far Hills, NJ: New Horizon Press.

This book shatters the stigma and shame that millions of men and women carry when their partners are sexually addicted. They receive little empathy for their pain, which means they suffer alone, often shocked and isolated by the trauma. Barbara Steffens' ground breaking new research shows that partners are not codependents but post-traumatic stress victims, while Marsha Means' personal experience provides insights, strategies, and critical steps to recognize, deal with, and heal partners of sexually addicted relationships. Firsthand accounts and stories reveal the impact of this addiction on survivors' lives.

Weiss, D. (2000). Steps to Freedom (2nd ed.). Colorado Springs, CO: Discovery Press.

This book follows the tradition of the Twelve Steps from a Christian perspective. It breaks down the various principles to help the reader experience freedom from sex addiction.

Weiss R. (2011). Cruise Control: Understanding Sex Addiction in Gay Men Robert Weiss ReadHowYouWant.

The author focuses on the clinical approach, asking the question, "Is your sexual behavior causing problems in other areas of your life?" Cruise Control leads men to a better understanding of the difference between sexual compulsion and non-addictive sexual behavior within the gay experience, and it explains what resources are available for recovery. Cruise Control provides understanding, empathy and encouragement to gay men seeking healthy sexual expression.

Weiss R.& Schneider, J. (2006). Untangling the Web: Sex, Porn, and Fantasy Obsession in the Internet Age. Boston MA: Alyson Books.

With personal stories from addicts and their significant others, this updated essential resource offers realistic healing strategies for anyone experiencing the devastating impact of Internet pornography and sex addiction on intimacy, relationships, career, health, and self-respect.

References

American Psychiatric Association, (2000): <u>Diagnostic and Statistical Manual of Mental Disorders.</u> (4th ed., Text Revision). Washington, D.C: American Psychiatric Association.

Arterburn, S., Stoeker, F., & Yorkey, M. (2000) <u>Every Man's Battle: Winning the War on Sexual Temptation One Victory at a Time</u>. Colorado Springs, CO: WaterBrook Press.

Beattie, M (1992). <u>Codependent No More: How to Stop Controlling Others and Start Caring for Yourself.</u> (2nd ed.). Center City, Mn: Hazelden.

Bradshaw, J. (1988). <u>Bradshaw On: The Family: A Revolutionary Way of Self-Discovery</u>. Deerfield Beach, FL: Health Communications, Inc.

Carnes, P. (1994). <u>Contrary to Love: Helping the Sexual Addict.</u> Minneapolis, MN: CompCare Publications, 1989.

Carnes, P. (1992). <u>Don't Call it Love: Recovery from Sexual Addiction</u>. New York: Bantam, 1991.

Carnes, P. (2001). <u>Out of the Shadows: Understanding Sexual Addiction.</u> Center City, MN: Hazelden.

Carnes, P. & Harkin, M. (2010). <u>Facing the Shadow: Starting Sexual and Relationship Recovery.</u> Carefree, AZ: Gentle Path Press.

Carriage House Psychotherapy. "Resources." <u>Kavod Addiction Recovery Centers</u>. http:// www.kavodrecovery.com/resources.asp (accessed February 28, 2012).

Covenant Eyes. (Last retrieved January 28, 2012). http://www.covenanteyes.com/

Family Safe Media. (Retrieved January 25, 2012). http://www.familysafemedia.com/ pornography_statistics.html

Ewald, R. (2003, May 13). Sexual Addiction. <u>AllPsych Journal,</u> http://allpsych.com/journal/ sexaddiction.html (Retrieved April 26, 2012)

Hastings, A.S. <u>Treating Sexual Shame: A New Map for Overcoming Dysfuntion, Abuse, and Addiction.</u> Northvale, NJ: Jason Aronson, 1998.

Henslin, E. (1991) <u>David and His Family Tree</u>. Chapter one in Secrets of Your Family Tree: Healing for Adult Children of Dysfunctional Families, by Dave Carder, Earl Henslin, John Townsend, Henry Cloud and Alice Brawand, 23-48. Chicago, IL: Moody.

Lerner, H. (1985). <u>The Dance of Anger: A Woman's Guide to Changing the Patterns of Intimate Relationships.</u> New York: Harper & Row.

Medinger, A. (1995, February). Accountability: Making it Work. <u>Regeneration News</u>

Schneider, J., Corley, M., & Irons, R.(1998). Surviving Disclosure of Infidelity: Results of an International Survey of 164 Recovering Sex Addicts and Partners. <u>Sexual Addiction & Compulsivity, 5,3,</u> 189-217.

Sexaholics Anonymous (1989) <u>SA Literature. Sexaholics Anonymous.</u>(1989). Nashville, TN.